Charming and earnest...an open-hearted and informative reflection on the experience of living with IBD.

—Jonathan Braun, MD, PhD
Professor and Chair
Pathology and Laboratory Medicine
UCLA David Geffen School of Medicine

Where was this book ten years ago when I needed it? When I was a freshman in college, I told my boyfriend that I had ulcerative colitis. Being the sensitive young man he was, he laughed and kept repeating, "Oh my god, you have bloody diarrhea? You have bloody diarrhea?"

I suppose it goes without saying that my feelings were quite bruised. If I had been armed with your book at the time I could have either clobbered him over the head with it or told him to read it and get a clue.

Colitiscope *is a practical resource and a self-esteem booster all wrapped into one.*

—Emily Sippola, RN, BAN
Minneapolis, Minnesota

As a parent, I have watched and experienced my son's struggles with Crohn's disease, but reading your words gives me a better understanding. I can really relate as a loved one.

I think this is a great book that has never been written before and should be on the reading list of everyone with IBD—to realize there is still life after diagnosis. This is very practical, and all ages will find parts they can identify with. It's a quick read with lots of humor and smiles.

—Carolyn Bloom, PT
Lawrence, Kansas

D1125411

ColitiScope

**Living with Crohn's Disease
and Ulcerative Colitis
Adventures · Humor · Insights**

Andrew Tubesing

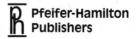
Pfeifer-Hamilton
Publishers

Pfeifer-Hamilton Inc, Publisher
Produced and distributed by Nordicom
Albuquerque, New Mexico
(866) 535-0222
www.colitiscope.net

Colitiscope: Living with Crohn's Disease and Ulcerative Colitis
Adventures • Humor • Insights

10 9 8 7 6 5 4 3 2 1

Printed in the United States of America by McNaughton & Gunn, Inc.
Printed on 100% post-consumer recycled paper and FSC-certified cover stock.

Copy Editor: Susan Rubendall
Artwork & Design: Joy Morgan Dey

Library of Congress Cataloging-in-Publication Data
2008941962

ISBN 978-1-935388-00-5

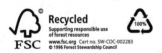

Recycled
Supporting responsible use
of forest resources
FSC www.fsc.org Cert no. SW-COC-002283
© 1996 Forest Stewardship Council
100%

*To my wife Heather
and my ever-supportive
friends and family*

*And to all supporters
of people with chronic conditions*

You are our heroes

*A portion of the proceeds from this book will be used
to support efforts that work toward curing IBD and
improving the lives of IBD patients.*

Table of Contents

Part II: Scope & Cope

Foreword

I have inflammatory bowel disease, also known as IBD. Mostly it appears to be ulcerative colitis, but some indicators suggest that I might have Crohn's disease. This book is the story of my life with colitis, from the initial discovery to the many resulting adventures that have followed. It offers perspectives on living with IBD and the laughs and tears it can bring.

There's no shortage of books that cover the clinical elements— the diagnosis, the details of the disease, the treatments and medications. But there are few publications that focus on the life this illness brings, the coping tools, the joy and sorrow. And there are even fewer that are funny. Call it the softer side, if you like, but after reading all the encyclopedic medical material, I was ready for the second act, the part about how to make life work in the midst of a chronic disease. From that gap grew my inspiration for this book. I can't promise you a foolproof solution, but I can give you a picture of what my life is like, and maybe that's a start.

If I had my way, IBD patients would read, enjoy, laugh, and learn from my experiences—and also share my insights with their family and friends as a way to help them understand what we go through. If I can articulate some of my quirky observations in a meaningful way that you can all enjoy, then I have accomplished my purpose.

In these pages you'll find funny stories, interesting tidbits, advice, insight, and much more. I have interspersed escapades with parables, and mixed in plenty of practical tips as well. I have also included information about common procedures, medications, and symptoms—but it will be unlike the stuff you've read elsewhere. Here I'll give you the straight talk, the inside scoop, and you will laugh, I promise. It's time to set your embarrassment aside and get out your funny bone.

The chapters are organized into two sections. Part I introduces the chronological development of my disease and associated adventures—which represents the "Colitis" side of Colitiscope. Part II explores the perspectives, life challenges, and solutions—making up the "Scope" and "Cope" portions of Colitiscope. From this collection, it is my hope that you will learn, share, and laugh.

❖ ❖ ❖

My wife, Heather, is the most patient person I've ever known, and I can never thank her enough for that and everything else. My parents have supported and encouraged me, instilling in me the tools I need to live a whole life. My brother, friends, colleagues, and others all make sacrifices which accommodate my illness (and strangeness, freakishness, and whatever else I may be). My doctors and advisors, my contacts at the Crohn's and Colitis Foundation of America (CCFA), and so many others have helped me to get where I am. I thank you all.

Part I

Colitis

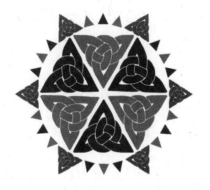

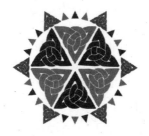

Bloody Bongiorno

It was about an hour before sunrise on earth, but perhaps only a few minutes before from my vantage point. Flying at 35,000 feet above Greenland, my brother, Phil, and I peered out the window of a 747. We were on our way to spend two weeks in Italy, France, and Spain with our parents and my wife, Heather. The northern lights were spectacular. Green and blue streaks of ghostly iridescence danced in the dawn sky, shimmering across a backdrop of stars and planets. It was a truly magical sight. We had been enroute for quite some time. We were landing in Amsterdam in a few hours then boarding another plane to Rome. It was the night before Christmas Eve, and we would spend it in Rome. As a family we had taken a Caribbean cruise together at Christmas time, but otherwise this was our first time spending the holidays away from home. We were all looking forward to it.

I normally experience some digestive trouble when I travel. There's nerves, there's getting up way too early in the morning to leave for the airport, and there's strange foods on an odd schedule. It all usually gives me a stomach ache and unpredictable bowels. I call it "travel tummy" as it's so common with air travel for me. But this time it was different. I had more than an unsettled stomach—it was more like an ache, like the kind you get before the flu. I wasn't nauseous at all, just troubled at the other end. I wrote it off as a worse-than-usual case of travel nerves.

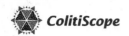

We landed in Amsterdam where we had a significant layover. With access to the airline's upscale travel club, we spent the idle time in style. Free champagne and food, nice environs, Internet access—and thankfully, nice bathrooms, because that's where I spent most of my time. I was hitting the toilet every fifteen minutes at that point. It wasn't very productive, just small amounts of quasi-solid waste, but it came out rather strangely, with an unusual kind of discomfort. Not pain exactly, just a sort of general unpleasant sensation, like passing a pine cone with the grain.

For travel tummy I could hardly have asked for better accommodations. The bathroom was immaculately clean, covered floor to ceiling in small white square tiles with solid brass faucets on elegant sinks and ivory glass light fixtures giving it a warm glow. The stalls were actually separate rooms walled in the same shiny tile with real solid wood doors. It was a lovely way to spend seven hours on the can, if such a thing is possible.

I was hoping for some sleep on the next flight, assuming my tummy would settle down as the travel demands eased up. No such luck. We arrived in Rome and took a taxi to the apartment we had rented for the week. It was just around the corner and a block down from Piazza Navonna. On arrival, out of necessity, I immediately familiarized myself with the bathroom. Our lodging was a cozy little academic pad with floor-to-ceiling bookshelves stocked with musty volumes, a small kitchen, and a couple of bedrooms. It was an old structure from a time before electricity so there was a vertical shaft through the middle of the building to which you could open windows in the kitchen and bathroom for light and ventilation.

We briefly explored the neighborhood, had a snack from the local deli, and went to bed. Finally I got some sleep. In the morning we went about exploring the area. It was Christmas eve, so by nightfall there were crowds of people out walking the narrow streets. Church bells were ringing everywhere, and it was generally festive.

My digestive system seemed to have gotten some relief from the night's rest, but it was still being rather unpredictable. The quasi-solids gave way to mostly-liquids. I was having a hard time finding menu items that seemed appealing—my system didn't want to ingest food that badly. I had no trouble salivating over the fresh chocolate crepes though; they were delicious. We also frequented the deli nearby, enjoying fresh baked breads, unbelievably good pesto, and thinly-sliced salami.

As we spent our days seeing the sights and absorbing the history, my system became increasingly agitated. Bathroom visits were more frequent and urgent and hardly ever solid anymore. They say Rome is the city of fountains—well there was an extra one in town that week. I gave some thought to renaming my backside Trevi. It's not always easy to find a bathroom in big cities, especially when you're linguistically challenged. I had taken a lot of Spanish classes, so that helped a little, but Italian is really quite different.

At some point my bathroom visits started getting painful. Sometimes it felt like my rectum was on fire. Was Nero's ghost still roaming around Rome? Had he somehow taken up in my back door? The episodes came and went, so I was able to be out and about enough to enjoy the visit, but my nerves were growing ever less comfortable with what I was experiencing.

My mood changed significantly, however, when I started to see blood in the toilet. Shifting from discomfort to serious concern, I immediately started to wonder what sort of bug I might have picked up over there, but remembered that the problems really started on the airplane. Planes are easy places to pick up viruses and other germs, but I wondered if any transmittable illness could have taken hold that quickly.

I remembered a former co-worker who once had rectal bleeding. Another colleague whose wife was a nurse commented on the situation, "That can mean a lot of things, but nothing good." Which left me with the impression that rectal bleeding is definitely bad news. I remember hearing about his doctor visit where they wanted to do some sort of test and him saying something like,

"You want to stick a *what* in my *where?* No way I'm gonna let you do that. Good bye."

He walked out and never went back. That was very much like him. He worked hard and had obvious carpel tunnel in his wrists, which bothered him all the time, but he would always be tough and shake things off. So it didn't surprise me that he might try to shake off the bleeding too. I never did learn what it was all about; he is not at all the sort of guy to talk about that with anyone, so I was left to assume the worst.

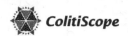

And now that it was happening to me, it made me nervous. I kept it to myself, though it was hard for others not to pick up on the frequency of my porcelain visitations. Heather remembers noticing my distress but claims that I didn't say anything about blood until we got home. I don't remember it that way, but it certainly could have been possible—I didn't even want to admit it to myself. Discovering a mysterious medical problem while traveling overseas was highly disconcerting. It was truly a bloody unwelcome welcome to Rome.

So I went about the trip trying to enjoy it as much as possible. But the digestive issues continued to develop.

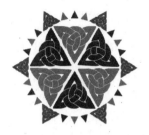

I Left My Underpants in Ancient France

I love boats more than just about anything—even more than I love macaroni and cheese, but not quite not as much as I love my wife. So I guess that's where they sit, number two on my romance list. Not surprisingly, Heather and I parted with the family after Rome and headed to Venice for its waterborne lifestyle. We spent over half of our two-week trip budget in just twenty-four hours, but it was worth every penny. Aside from enjoying all the great shopping and a ridiculously ornate Venetian glass chandelier in our hotel room (it literally occupied the entire ceiling), we rode on four different kinds of boats and saw all kinds of others, including a rickety old skiff with an outboard motor, piled high with a mountain of DHL overnight packages. Conditions in my belly were still just developing at this point, so I didn't have terrible bathroom trouble there, but that all changed once we got to France.

We rented a car in Nice and meandered our way through Provence to meet up with my brother in Avignon a few days later. The three of us would later rejoin my folks in Barcelona at week's end. However, there was some confusion about meeting Phil at the train station as planned because he didn't appear to get off the TGV train from Rome like he was supposed to. We waited a while

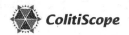

and worried that for some reason his plans had changed. Our pre-arranged agreement was to communicate by email if such a thing were to happen. So Heather and I decided to split up. She would stay and wait for him while I went to town in search of an Internet café. I got directions and headed out to the parking lot.

There I encountered one of those stressful occasions in which situations that appear familiar are actually completely different in a new culture. I got in the rental car and made my way to the parking lot exit. As I would expect with a pay lot in the states, I drove to the exit gate to pay for my time and be on my way. Well, there was no attendant at the exit, instead just a vending machine of some sort, but it had no coin slot, and the paper feeder didn't match the size of any of the French bills I had accumulated. There were some instructions—but all in French, though I recognized the word "sortie" as exit which was an encouraging find. The rest of what I stood a chance of comprehending was all in symbolic pictures. After a lot of staring, turning my head sideways, diagramming the activities pictured, (and some honking from cars behind me in line), I realized that the three or four icons I was gazing at ostensibly were meant to be the international language for "Before leaving the train station, guess at your parking duration, pay money into a vending machine inside the station, and bring the dispensed ticket here to get out." Brilliant. I was suddenly reminded of a college history professor who constantly chided the French throughout history. He would set up a dramatic story, which at some point would climax with something like "…and guess who was there to screw it all up? FRRRANCE!" He would growl loudly enough to wake sleeping students in adjacent classrooms.

For a moment I considered driving right through the gate in front of me. I looked in the rearview mirror and saw several cars waiting behind me. I checked the side mirrors and realized that we were all being funneled into this lane by curbs on both sides leading back at least three car lengths, penning us in. Turning back to the machine, scowling, I gave it "the finger," thus communicating the international symbol for "Why not put the stupid payment machine out here instead of inside the train station?"

I looked in the mirror again, signaling to the guy behind me that he needed to back up and let me out. I put the car in reverse, hoping the back-up lights would give him a clue. He honked, and I could see he was making international symbols of his own. I waved him back. He motioned behind him like he was stuck, making a point of showing his irritated expression. At this point, I finally tried to get out of the car so I could signal the drivers behind him that I am an American idiot who needs everybody to back up because I don't know their backward rules. Instead I got pinched in the door because it hit the machine and wouldn't open far enough to let me out. I writhed around for a few seconds until finally someone got the idea and the cars started backing out to let me finish embarrassing myself.

I parked again and went back inside the train station to buy a parking ticket. Actually I didn't mind it much at that point because my rear end was signaling that it was ready for a sortie of its own. I briefly wondered again why I was having all these urgent bathroom visits and took care of that need first, then found the parking ticket kiosk. I had no idea how much time to pay for, so I bought the most expensive option, which I assumed was an all day pass—it might have been a penny or a hundred bucks, I had no idea, the French money had only been in my pocket for a day or two, so I hadn't yet adapted to the conversion.

This time I successfully exited the parking lot and made my way to old town where I was told I could find Internet access. After a moderate hassle parking on the street and dealing with a parking meter, I logged on at a café and found no email from my brother. I sent him a message saying we would wait at the train station and check email every two hours until we heard something.

On my way back I encountered a less-than-delightful maze of one-way streets. Approaching the station I accidentally chose the wrong ramp and had to circle back. Finally I returned and searched the terminal for Heather. I found her sipping coffee with my brother in a pair of lounge chairs, drenched in morning sun streaming through the glass wall behind them. Contrary to my disposition at the time, they looked relaxed, almost bored. Then I heard the wonderful news. Turns out he was on the train after all, and she found him only a couple minutes after we split up. Yep, before I humiliated myself in the parking lot, before I came in for the bathroom and the

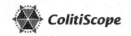

parking ticket, before I even went into town. Ugh. *Hopefully this day will get better,* I thought to myself. Well, it didn't.

Heather and Phil both studied French in high school, so as we headed for the parking lot, they bought the parking ticket this time— paying considerably less money than I did. On the way out of town we stopped at a suburban shopping center for some lunch. Because I visit hardware stores everywhere I travel, no matter what, we also stopped at the French version of Home Depot, where I couldn't resist buying some light fixtures to mail home (which I have yet to install, of course).

Our primary destination was Carcassonne, an old city near the Spanish border whose fortifications date back to Roman times. It is a beautiful ancient city, all of which is old by our standards, but the really old part is the hilltop inner fortress, which is only accessible on foot. We spent a lovely afternoon exploring the stone walls and cobblestone pathways. We shopped and gazed at the architecture. While perusing the Basilica's cavernous interior, after eating something with a forgettable name (but an entirely memorable result), I felt the inklings of a bathroom call. Inklings quickly turned to pestering, and I suddenly had an emergency on my hands. Oh wow, it was bad. I signaled to Heather and Phil that I needed a bathroom, quick. We all looked around, there didn't appear to be anything inside the sanctuary. One of them asked a docent, "Le somethingorother merci…" who pointed us outside and up the pathway to a public restroom.

I hurried outside, but by the time I could see my destination I was pretty sure it was already too late. I scrambled up the street to some stone steps leading down into the bathroom. It had a Gothic arched doorway, and the floor was paved with large chunks of stone, worn in by the ages. Dark and cavernous like a dungeon, the only light inside streamed in through slits in the rock wall high above me. Some horribly out-of-place modular restroom wall dividers sectioned off a stall in the middle of the open room with urinals to the left, sinks to the right. I was really crowning by then, and as I entered the stall some gas escaped. Or so I thought, but it wasn't just gas, too wet for that. I didn't even have my pants down yet. Crap!

Inside the stall, much to my chagrin, I found a Turkish toilet. A Turkish toilet is less like a toilet and more like a hole in the floor.

I didn't even know they had them in France. *I was in Carcassonne after all,* I reminded myself. *Some of it was built during the Ottoman Empire; perhaps this bathroom still had some original fixtures.* The toilet was made of stone or clay and resembled a urinal, turned on its back and recessed in the floor. Apparently I was supposed to straddle this thing, balancing in a squat position with my pants around my ankles while trying not to fall over or soil myself. But it appeared as though I had already done that. It was also apparent that a previous visitor didn't like the toilet any more than I did and had decided not to use it. There was crap on the floor in the corner, literally. It smelled awful, though it also seemed perfectly fitting for the medieval context. I breathed through my mouth to minimize the stench.

I carefully took down my pants as quickly as I could, and before I even finished squatting the juice was flowing. This episode was rather painful, coming out in spasms, sort of like when you vomit. I was in a large stall; the walls were spaced wide enough that I could not reach them from the middle. As I crouched precariously with nothing within reach to aid my balance, I inspected my pants. My boxers had suffered damage, but I couldn't find any remnants elsewhere. I could see that it indeed was not just gas that snuck out; instead it was mostly blood with some other not-so-appealing substances mixed in. I turned to look at what I'd let out behind me, but couldn't make the contortion to bring it into view. I shuffled my feet and turned a bit to see that it was indeed bloody and yucky. *What does this mean?* I wondered quietly. I swallowed the panic, reassuring myself that I'd be home in a week, and if it hadn't stopped by then I would see a doctor. With the circulation cut off at my knees, my feet were going numb. Squatting is not a natural position for me. The last thing I needed was to fall backward into my own mess.

It seemed as though I was finished so I looked around for some toilet paper—and that's when my day really took a downhill turn. There wasn't any paper, but it wasn't because they had run out. Rather I saw absolutely no evidence of there ever having been toilet paper there, not even a dispenser. The history professor's voice echoed in my head, *"FRRRANCE!"* Now this was not current-day France; there was no cute little butt-shower there either. Carcassonne was built long before the advent of Prissy-Pants France. I

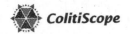

don't know when the bidet was conceived, but if they never figured out the toilet paper thing, I guess I can't really blame them for its invention.

My knees were burning by then so I had to stand up. I could feel a couple drops of blood falling free as I raised up to a quasi-erect, bent-over position, keeping my knees bent slightly, ensuring some overhang to protect my clothes. I braced my hands on my knees and took a deep breath. It stunk. *What do I do now?* I puzzled. I had nothing but a postcard in my pocket. I looked down again at my underwear. Could they be revived? I pondered the situation for a long moment. My legs started trembling slightly from fatigue, telling me I needed to figure it out soon. Then it hit me. I could take my boxers off, use the unsoiled parts to clean myself up, and then throw them away. *Oh man. Oh man!* My heart sank in painful agony as I considered what I had to do. I am sure the look on my face reflected the disgusting situation I was in and the tragedy I was about to inflict upon myself.

Now hold that picture of my expression in your mind for a moment. This is the part in a movie where the screen freeze-frames on the protagonist's face while he is enduring some egregious hardship and making a bizarre expression. We get an extended look at that face while he narrates some back story that makes sense of what you are about to witness. We get snapshots of these past moments. In this case, he (I) says,

Now let me tell you something. I love my underwear. Maybe not as much as boats or my wife, but it's certainly up there with mac and cheese. And these weren't any old underwear, these were precious...irreplaceable.

Finding good underwear is a painstaking and expensive process. It takes a few tries before you find the ones that will work for the long haul, then you go back and get more. Well the ones I wear now I had discovered about 8 years ago. They're simple cotton knit boxers, but instead of the bulky bunched-together elastic waistband common to most standard boxer shorts, these have some stretchy Lycra in the fabric, and the top edge is simply folded over and sewn down in a two-inch hem, making for a very low-profile and comfy waist. There's nothing else like it on the market. When I first found them, I fell in love. I bought a sufficient supply and went on with life. At the time I was working on a nationwide publicity tour and lived on the road for nine months straight. When I returned home and readjusted to normal life, I went back to Penneys to stock up on my magic underwear. But I couldn't find it. I searched everywhere. Finally I asked a clerk where they were.

"Do you mean those Jockey Zone boxers?" She asked.

"Yes, those are the ones."

"Oh they were discontinued a couple months ago, we won't be getting any more."

"You mean discontinued by the manufacturer, or did you just stop carrying them?" I asked.

"No they stopped making them."

My jaw dropped. I couldn't believe my ears. Not again. It seems like every product I come to love inevitably gets discontinued. Friends and family make fun of me for how product-loyal I can be. I am the world's most harsh product critic, but when I find something that's perfect, I am a subscriber for life. When they discontinued my deodorant, I called the company and ordered a full case of it from their backstock. People said it wouldn't last, it would evaporate, but they were wrong. Last year I finished the last of it after rationing it out to myself for more than a decade. Yes I'm a freak. In fact, on this very trip to France I had rediscovered my old favorite shaving gel, which had been discontinued in the states, so I was thrilled to see it still available in Europe, and I bought more everyplace I saw it. My brother, who travels a lot, was still bringing it to me up to a couple years ago. But none of us can find it anymore, even overseas—or on eBay. (I am nearly out now, if you have some or know where to get it, please send it to me care of the publisher. It's called Gillette Shaving Concentrate and comes in a silver oblong ribbed plastic bottle, SKU#50785896. I will reward you handsomely.)

I was furious. *That was the best underwear ever made, how could they stop making it?* I started breathing heavily. The clerk stared at me. My peripheral vision started going fuzzy, then dark. I could see only a blurry circle in front of me. I walked away from the counter. Turning down the maze of department store aisles, I navigated with foggy tunnel vision. When I got back to the car I had to take some deep breaths and calm myself down before driving home.

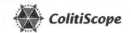

I guess it is sort of funny looking back, but I certainly wasn't amused at the time. Later I told a friend about it. She knew how much I loved my undies and understood the tragedy, but she laughed anyway. Fair enough, I always laughed at her because her family called underwear "chuds." Perhaps now you'll understand how angry I was when I found the waistband of one of these boxers in the backyard crap of my roommate's dog. It was bad enough being out there poop-scooping, but to find that the dog had shredded and eaten a pair of my priceless shorts added significant insult. In any case, the tragedy is now tempered by the fact that boxers are simply incompatible with inflammatory bowel disease for obvious practical reasons. Like it or not, I didn't need them any more.

So back to Carcassonne, the cameras are rolling again. There I stood in ancient France wearing irreplaceable underpants. The world's supply of these boxers was down to eleven, and I was preparing to obliterate nine percent of the stockpile in one fell swoop. Not to mention, on a long trip losing a pair of chuds has a significant impact on laundry planning. I hated to admit it to myself; I cringed at the thought, but I knew what I must do. Easier said than done, however.

As I mentioned earlier, there was already somebody else's scat on the floor, and who knows what else had been there. I was going to have to remove my shoes and extract my undies from my pants and legs without smearing anything on myself or dripping anything from my bum. I slowly pried each shoe off, standing on top of them. I held my boxers at mid-thigh spreading my knees enough to keep them taut and elevated, while carefully working my jeans off by stepping on each cuff with the other foot and wiggling my legs out. With the precision of that buzzing Operation game from my childhood, I raised each foot through the leg holes of my shorts without touching them on the way out. Somehow I succeeded in keeping myself clean throughout this delicate procedure. I meticulously wrapped and folded the boxers as I turned them into the world's most precious ass wipe. It pained me to treat them this way, but I had no choice. I set them on the floor and carefully re-dressed, being sure not to track nasty bathroom floorness onto my socks and into my shoes. I would have to finish the day commando style. If nature were to make another emergency call I would be in big trouble. *Better not eat anything until we find our hotel,* I concluded.

I waited to be sure there was no one else in the bathroom and emerged from the stall with my tragedy in hand, heading straight for the trash can. I said goodbye to the yucky bundle, looking at it one more time before I let the spring-loaded cover close over the can. I washed my hands about seventeen times, double-checked my clothes for unwanted remnants, and headed back into the light.

Ascending from the dungeon, I found Heather and Phil sitting on a short section of stone wall chatting about something. I had been gone a long time. Heather gave me a concerned look, and Phil just sat there patiently, looking ready to move on. This would be the beginning of a very unusual relationship for them. Everywhere we went, from that point forward, the two of them would be left to entertain themselves while I ran for the toilet. We travel together a lot, so over the years I suspect they've had hundreds of these chats. I wonder what they talk about all that time, which of the world's problems they could solve while I'm in the can. They could probably write a book to describe their side of the adventures we share from opposite sides of bathroom walls.

Diagnosed / Be Prepared

Upon returning to the states from those two weeks in Europe, during which time my situation had evolved from a simple tummy ache to incessant diarrhea and bloody stools, I made a beeline for the doctor.

I first saw a nurse practitioner at my family physician's office. I had seen a doctor for hemorrhoids once a number of years previous and received a taste of the awkwardness of confessing and surrendering to inspection of problems in such a personal location. But that visit was relatively simple—just a quick slice with a scalpel, and it was over. This time, we shared several long minutes of probing with a track & field relay baton (the sterile version of which is called a proctoscope). It's a rigid hollow pipe about an inch thick that allows inspection of the rectum and lower sigmoid colon.

After a bit of spelunking around with a flashlight, she concluded quite readily that I needed a more sophisticated evaluation. She said I definitely had some inflammation and that I'd need to see the local surgeon for a colonoscopy so they could determine the extent of my problem. After a bunch of questions and explanations, they called and got me an appointment. The procedure seemed simple enough except for two things. First, it required sedation, which meant I had to come with someone to drive me home. Second, it was to be performed in an operating room. OK, in my book, nothing that requires an O.R. and a chaperone is a casual affair. I was definitely curious,

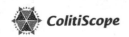

if not mostly nervous. To me, it seemed like a procedure that fancy must mean bad news. But at least I was finally getting help for my mysterious problem; most of the previous weeks on vacation had been pretty nerve-racking.

Before I left the office, the staff gave me a bunch of papers describing what I had to do to get ready for the colonoscopy. Instructions for preparation were lengthy and required that I obtain some supplies from the pharmacy, notably a bottle of Fleet Phospho-soda (a liquid laxative) and a plethora of fluids—everything from apple juice to beef broth.

I so enjoy the concept they refer to as "preparation." This is one of those government-style euphemisms where they try to make a fifty-ton bomb sound like a firecracker. I know what that's all about; the university where I work has a division that specializes in explosives testing, which they so delicately refer to as "Energetic Materials Research."

The purpose of preparation is to empty your system of any and all food remains. They want a perfectly clear view of your insides when they shove that six-foot hose up your porthole. If there's anything still in the intestine it can get in the way or be mistaken for problems, so they advise eating nothing red for a couple days (sorry kids, no beets tonight!). Then you get only clear liquids for the last twenty-four hours and nothing for the final six or so, not even water. Obviously there's a reason the GI procedure lab has a "no food or drink" policy, even for visitors. It's to stop those thoroughly prepared folks from causing riots in the waiting room.

The day before my procedure I got out my bottle of Fleet Phospho, read the directions, referred back to the doctor's instructions one last time, and started swigging away. Now that was an education. I quickly learned that the real meaning of preparation is drinking between a quart and a gallon of this vile seawater solution, which within the hour, comes out the other end as the entire Pacific Ocean. Talk about energetic materials, wow! I think I had enough rocket boost to put the space shuttle in orbit. If there were a way to harness this hydropower, we could solve the energy crisis—then people would be running around talking about how cool it is to have colitis. But at the time I had no idea how "cool" I was destined to become.

When they say "prepared," they *really* mean prepared. I mean *everything* empties out—breakfast, lunch, and dinner, yesterday's spinach salad, last night's hot wings (ouch)...even the matchbox car you swallowed at Billy Zinkewicz's seventh birthday party, and all that gum you ate in junior high. I swear if I'd still had an appendix it would have come out too.

This process brings new meaning to the Boy Scout motto, "Be prepared," only in this case it feels less like something one does voluntarily and more like something that is done to them, "to be prepared," sort of like to be robbed, or invaded, or served, or subpoenaed...glamorous indeed. The Fleet Phospho should come with a free T-shirt that says "I've Been Prepared" with their logo under it. But somehow I don't think they're going to be marketing to the general consumer any time soon. Another of the preparation laxatives they sometimes use is called Golytely, which is a gallon jug of 100 percent pure irony.

Funny that the two days of preparation would seem like the easy part, which it definitely is not. It's forty-eight hours of misery all to get ready for a fifteen-minute procedure. Then it's suddenly over.

Anyway, on colonoscopy day my nervous wait continued at the hospital where I was assigned a room to get ready and to which I would be returning later for recovery. A nurse came in to start my IV. She picked up on my anxiety and offered me something to calm me down. I declined—I thought I would be having enough medications that day as it was. I waited about fifteen minutes in the bed with Heather sitting by my side. Finally they came to take me to the O.R. Heather stayed behind and read her book.

The operating room looked pretty calm, though I was definitely not feeling calm. The nurse anesthetist talked me through what we were about to do together. I asked some questions, mostly wanting to know what it would feel like and what the drugs would do to me. Of everything going on, the medication was the scariest part for me. Drugs that transport a person to La-La Land make me nervous. Plus, after doing some reading on the topic, I realized that a good portion of the risk in this procedure is with the drugs themselves. What they used was basically a strong sedative that would relax me and suppress my memory, without really putting me to sleep. After

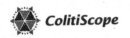

a few minutes of hooking me up to various machines, he shot a syringe-full into my IV tube and I drifted off.

The procedure was performed by a general surgeon. I learned later that this is relatively unusual. These days, colonoscopies are typically performed by gastroenterologists (doctors who specialize in the digestive system). However, since I lived in a small community isolated in the desert southwest, relatively distant from the nearest specialist, this surgeon was the only qualified colonoscopy practitioner in town.

One of the books I read later contained an interesting comment. It was trying to reassure the reader that, while partially conscious during sedation, you won't say embarrassing things; this must be a concern for some patients I guess. I couldn't take that as anything but a bunch of hooey though, because of my memory of this colonoscopy experience. I woke up speaking Spanish to the nurse. I have no idea what I was saying, but much of the Spanish that I remember is not the sort of stuff you say in front of decent company. Nearly everybody speaks Spanish in New Mexico, so I'm sure at least half the room knew what I was saying—I only wish I knew myself. It must have been either funny or embarrassing because I do remember them chuckling at something I said, but I was pretty woozy, so it's a vague memory at best.

They wheeled me back into the hospital room to regain my senses. I found Heather waiting for me there. The surgeon had already stopped by to explain everything to her. As I re-oriented myself, she described what he had said. I remembered very little of it later so she had to repeat it again. We spent about an hour there while I drank fluids and finished waking up, and then they let me go. I was a little disappointed that the surgeon never came back to explain it all to me personally, but Heather had gotten the word so I guess they figured that was good enough.

He had told her that I had colitis, an inflammation of the colon that could be mitigated with medication. He showed her some pictures taken during the procedure with the fiber-optic scope camera, and explained a little about what he saw. She did her best to translate it to me later, but there wasn't a lot of information to go on.

I went in for a follow-up a few days later. That is where I got the colitis diagnosis personally. But, as I would come to learn later, the surgeon did a terrible job of explaining it. He told me basically the same thing he'd told Heather after my procedure. It was an inflammation of the colon, and I should take Asacol and come back in a month.

This all sounded simple enough. Sort of like strep throat or a sinus infection. Take these meds and come back for a check-up. So I took the Asacol as directed, and my symptoms resolved in a couple of weeks. After a month I saw the surgeon again, and he cleared me to stop taking the meds. Another follow-up a month later got me fully discharged from his care without any fanfare or warnings—in fact no indication at all that there was anything to worry about.

Piece of cake. At no point during any of this was I given the impression that it was anything other than a quick-fix problem. So I didn't worry about it much, and I went on with life. I had a busy summer planned and started preparing for my upcoming projects.

* * *

A note on the colonoscopy experience before we move on: I have since had several more of these procedures, but I've never used sedation again. I did some research on the topic and found that using sedation as a routine part of the procedure is much more common in America than anywhere else. Most other places around the world don't use it, and consider it unnecessary except in cases of extreme discomfort. The reasoning is, as I said earlier, that the medication introduces an additional level of risk. Very rarely the colon can be perforated by one of the instruments, which requires emergency surgery, but problems with the sedatives also occur which increase the total risk of complications.

Another disadvantage of being sedated is that it extends the recovery time. On following occasions, when I declined the sedatives, I was able to get off the bed, get dressed, and go home—instead of spending an hour in recovery and a queasy day or so of expelling the drugs from my system.

The most important part about staying awake for the colonoscopy is that it gives you a whole new understanding about your condition—with the ability to watch and track your progress yourself with your own eyes—and a new language to discuss it. You can talk with the doctor as it's happening, and he or she can explain what they see and what it means. And it's truly interesting to see what it all looks like inside.

So, given these factors, why is the use of sedation still so popular in America? First, I suspect that medical professionals prefer to sedate patients because they are easier to work with. Second, it offers the patient a way to escape the embarrassing process of being worked on in a private area. To me, the drugs are not worth it, but some people would rather not be conscious. Regardless of your preference, understand that you do have a choice, and it's one you can research and consider for yourself.

One thing that gave me the confidence to decline sedatives during my second colonoscopy is that I'd had several sigmoidoscopy procedures prior to it. A sigmoidoscopy is a miniature colonoscopy done in the gastroenterologist's office. The scope goes in about half as far, and it only takes a few minutes. I typically don't need to prepare for this one, and there's no sedation involved, so it's sort of a warm-up to the biggie.

It seems like allowing such a personal inspection would be embarrassing, but it's a lot easier if you realize that they do this all day, every day. These procedures we're not accustomed to experiencing are things they do all the time, so they understand what you're going through and take measures to ease your awkwardness.

If you are inclined to try a colonoscopy without sedation, it may be difficult to convince the procedure team that you really want to (or can) do it. It's a pretty unusual request, and they generally don't like to do it that way. But I insist on it when I go, and it's really not that difficult for me. You'll have an IV in your arm anyway, so they can administer the meds during the procedure if you find you want or need them. I once had a colonoscopy team confess afterward that they'd put wagers on whether I would make it through without sedation. I think most of them lost money betting against me.

If the team talks you into doing the colonoscopy sedated, you'll miss all the fun and just wake up farting in the recovery room. During the procedure, you may be observant and conversational, but it's likely that you won't remember it. That's why staying fully awake for this procedure is so valuable—it allows you to see firsthand what your symptoms look like, and remember it all. And that's worth it to me. On the other hand, upper endoscopy (the one that goes down your throat) is a bit more difficult without sedation, despite the anti-gag throat-numbing spray (make sure they use a lot of it). The other bummer with this procedure is you really can't watch it because you and the doctor are not facing the same direction.

Reprise / Surprise

Given the fact that this is a book about colitis and living a life that includes it, perhaps it's obvious to you that there has been no quick fix for me. Instead, over many years I have struggled to understand and cope with this disease. In the beginning, I never expected the problem to be long-term. Indeed I thought it was over after the original episode, but of course it was not. I was to discover that all too quickly.

Later in the summer after the first episode, maybe three months after finishing the initial treatment, my symptoms began to return once again. I found some familiar mucous in my stool, and I was getting a bit uncomfortable much like that day spent in the Amsterdam airport.

I was traveling at the time, on rounds doing work for old clients, updating systems, and adding new ones—my typical summer contracting work in Midwestern farm country. My wife and I had both grown up in northern Minnesota, and only recently moved to the Southwest, so I still had work contacts in the region. One of the projects required me to add a wireless data link from a college campus to a hospital annex across town. I was working on the roof of the highest building in town, a twelve-story dormitory atop the only significant hill for miles—a convenient high point for the whole county. As a result, this roof served as an antenna farm for all sorts of communications technology—cellular phones, pagers, two-way

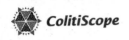

radio systems for businesses, police, and fire departments, etc. I had to take the elevator to the top floor, walk up the stairs to the elevator equipment penthouse above, then climb a ladder up to the top roof to mount the antenna.

One day while working on that roof, I had my most significant indicator that the disease had returned. Absolutely out of the blue, with the urgency of a flash flood, I had to go the bathroom RIGHT NOW. Ohh man, I scrambled down the ladder and sped down the steps to the floor below. The dorm was unoccupied during the summer so I didn't need to worry about whether it was a men's or women's floor; I just made way for the nearest bathroom. Luckily I found a stall that still had a few remnants of toilet paper.

I made it down in time, but I sat there contemplating my situation, alone in this huge echo-ey bathroom atop a building that had been vacant for a month. It was one of my lonelier moments. Much was flooding through my mind (and bowels). I remember imagining a cascade of unpleasant thoughts. *This feels exactly like what I'd experienced in Europe a few months ago—a very similar progression from odd symptoms to extremely urgent bowel movements. Ugh, could this really be happening again? I thought this was all fixed up. Will these emergency poops keep happening? How am I supposed to work on the roof with this going on? Not only that, but the other end of this wireless link is atop a fifty-foot tower that I have to climb and strap myself on to...there's no way I'll be able to get down from there in time if this happens again.*

My heart was racing. Not only for the practical concerns, but for the larger issue of what the return of these symptoms might mean. *Why did this come back? Come to think of it, why did I get it in the first place?* The surgeon never really did explain that. And to my own discredit, I had never bothered to look it up myself. However, he didn't make colitis sound like a big deal, so it didn't occur to me that I should do any research.

I turned to look in the toilet and found that the only symptom missing this time was blood. But I reminded myself that came a little later last time, so it may still be on its way.

I sat there for a long time contemplating both how I would finish the work I was doing, and how this new development would affect my summer. I had projects to finish, some recreation planned, and a long road trip to get home in a few weeks. And my home doctor was fifteen hundred miles away.

I was able to finish that day's work without further incident, but I was definitely not relaxed. I'd been staying with a good friend in town who did similar work, so we'd been spending a lot of time together. He had split up with his longtime girlfriend the previous night. Being Friday, we were both ready to relax a bit, and considering both of our challenged emotional states at the time, we decided to get out of town for the weekend. We went to my folks' cabin a few hours away for a little R & R. It is located on a lake nestled in the north woods of Wisconsin; just the sort of retreat we were looking for.

My symptoms did not improve, and indeed the blood had returned by the next day. I was fairly well convinced the colitis had come back. But I was far from home and would be there for another month, so I needed to figure out what to do. I got on the Internet to see what I could learn about colitis. Nothing had prepared me for the surprise I was about to encounter. Everything I read about colitis on the web referred to it as a chronic illness. *Chronic, like permanent?* I wondered what they could be talking about. My doctor never made any comments to me about this being a chronic disease, or even the slightest bit serious condition. *Are they talking about the same thing? Couldn't be.* I kept looking but found nothing about any sort of casual, curable colitis and everything about incurable, life-long ulcerative colitis.

I called my cousin who is a physician. He confirmed that colitis is typically chronic, although some do get it and cure it without return, but that's quite rare.

The following Monday I called to inquire with the surgeon who had diagnosed me. I got a call back later in the day and he confirmed that it can be a chronic illness. However, he said that since mine went away so easily, he didn't consider it serious. Still I thought he should have at least alerted me to the fact that the chronic version was a possibility (if not a serious likelihood)!

I don't remember at which point I told Heather or what her reaction was. I was pretty angry and confused. I called my parents and my dad suggested an excellent internal medicine specialist in our old hometown not far away. With some coercion, I was able to get an appointment that Friday.

After some discussion and questioning, that doctor thought it was pretty obvious that I had ulcerative colitis, as I feared. He too was shocked that the initial diagnosing surgeon had made no mention of the potential seriousness. He also made it clear that I should really be seeing a gastroenterologist—a digestive disease specialist to whom I probably should have been referred upon my original diagnosis. The immediate solution would be to re-start the Asacol. Later, when I got home, I would see a proper gastroenterology (GI) specialist. The surgeon agreed with this plan and referred me to a GI clinic. I got an appointment for the week I was to return home.

The rest of that summer was pretty unpleasant. Symptoms persisted despite taking Asacol, which had worked so effectively and quickly before. My trepidation about having a chronic illness was really stressful. I was traveling alone for an extended time, not having much fun at all anymore. Heather was just a phone call away, but it felt like I was in a different world, somewhere far away and very lonely. I basically focused on getting my work done and hurrying home.

Upon my return to our southwest home, the appointment with the gastroenterologist was both relieving and disappointing. On that day, he performed my first sigmoidoscopy. I didn't really know what that was, but I quickly found out.

Being incredibly familiar with it by now, I have come to call it an *ass-spection*. A doctor magically finds a way to stuff two feet of three-eighths-inch hose into your nether area. It's basically a video game in which the doc uses a fiber-optic camera to explore a world unknown to all but the extremely lucky, which is displayed in real-time on a TV screen. With his scope he travels down soggy passageways while dodging bad guys called Stools. There are controls for the camera, lights, and windshield washer fluid, and there's even a robotic arm used for bringing moon rocks home. If the Stools are really ornery, the doctor gets rewarded with inflation privileges, pumping the colon full of air for easier navigation. And then you (and the people around you) get the unfriendly pleasure of the deflation process for the next few hours as the air finds its way out.

We both saw inflammation quite similar to what I'd seen in the colonoscopy photos. The colon, instead of looking pink and veiny, looked red and irritated, as if it had been rubbed with sandpaper. And there were little white ulcers all over the place, sort of like the marbling in a raw rib-eye steak. The inflammation went most of the way up my sigmoid colon, not quite to the transverse. That means about forty centimeters or so of nasty-looking irritation, the worst of which was in the rectum and lower sigmoid.

He was convinced that I had ulcerative colitis, the chronic condition I had come to fear. What a bummer.

"An incurable illness? How did I get it? Why? What do you do about it?" I had a lot of questions. He had some answers, but he wasn't much for conversation. Very clinical and minimal in his responses, he left me quite unenlightened. We upped my dosage of Asacol and made a follow-up appointment.

Asacol is a brand name for the drug mesalamine. It has anti-inflammatory properties similar to aspirin, and is somehow chemically related. It comes in the form of a time-release capsule that is designed to distribute its active ingredient when the pill reaches the colon, thus delivering the drug to the affected area. This drug also comes under different names in suppository and enema form. It had worked for me after the initial diagnosis, but this time it seemed to do nothing at all.

Two months later when I saw him again, there had been no improvement. In fact, my urgent bathroom visits were getting worse. We upped the Asacol dosage again. By the next visit I had developed increased pain and a condition called tenesmus (which can be a sort of dry-heaving at the rear end). So we scheduled a colonoscopy to get a better impression and take some biopsies.

The colonoscopy is basically a "sigmoidoscopy squared," but in this case it's a six-foot hose, and it can reach all the way to your small intestine. Also, don't forget, you get the true joy of 'preparation' for this one. You get to see tunnels and caves unlike those in the junior procedure. Plus if you're lucky you'll get to see your appendix, but I got ripped off on that because mine had already been removed (more on that later).

This colonoscopy was my first without sedation and I am very glad I did it that way. I got to see the entire process and understand what was going on. It was a little strange for me to watch them tear off biopsy samples with a little needle-nose extension, but I didn't feel anything. (This part of the process is typically painless because the surface layers of the intestinal wall have no nerves, but it is common to experience gas pains during the procedure.) Again though, this doctor did not communicate well. After the procedure he tried to explain the answers to my questions but I felt like I was like talking to a robot. He had little respect for the emotional side of my reactions. He treated everything as if it were routine, and provided no information that Heather and I didn't specifically ask for. It was frustrating to say the least.

The biopsy came back specifying inflammation consistent with ulcerative colitis, so I was pretty sure I didn't have to worry about Crohn's disease, which was a relief. Crohn's is the other half of inflammatory bowel disease. It is a cousin to ulcerative colitis with similar biological mechanisms and symptoms, but it is not limited to affecting the colon. It can spring up anywhere in the digestive tract and is therefore more invasive and more difficult to treat.

I read about the medications and treatments and wondered what would be next for me if Asacol continued to be ineffective. I was becoming more certain that this gastroenterologist was anything but effective for me. Over the next six months we kept fumbling around with Asacol. My symptoms kept getting worse, and I was becoming pretty miserable. And the bathroom visits! Ugh, they were completely dominating my life. Afraid to ever be more than fifteen seconds from the can, I could hardly go anywhere, especially after eating. Our grad-student lodger once commented that I perfectly demonstrated the Continuity Equation. This is a scientific law relating to the conservation of mass; for any process "mass in equals mass out." My body had a habit of balancing that equation quite rapidly.

By this time I had digested much clinical information from all the common sources. I had bought and read every book I could find on ulcerative colitis, Crohn's disease, and inflammatory bowel disease. At the time I didn't know there were IBD support groups, so I didn't seek out that option, though in hind sight I know that it would have helped me a great deal.

Around this time, however, I was able to make a personal connection with another IBD patient. I learned of a friend's cousin who had ulcerative colitis in college. It was the first time I'd encountered anyone else with the disease, and I eagerly contacted him for more information and a personal perspective, which was very helpful. Mostly it was nice to talk to an experienced patient. I started to feel a little less alone, knowing that there are others out there experiencing the same things. It was a great comfort.

His case had progressed quickly and was too severe for any of the available meds to help him. After less than a year of misery, he had a colectomy and the J-pouch surgery. Technically called an ileo-anal anastamosis, in this procedure the surgeons first remove the entire colon and rectum. Then they fashion a pouch by folding the last foot of the small intestine over itself (in a 'J' shape) and sew it together. Finally, the pouch is re-attached to the anus and serves as a replacement for the large intestine—a quasi-colon if you will.

This is a colectomy method that eliminates the need for an external ostomy bag to collect stool (except for a temporary intermediate period during the two-surgery process). For many recipients, relatively normal bowel function is restored, though stools are never truly solid anymore. People can live without their colon because its main purposes are to extract salt and water from the stool and to serve as a storage reservoir. Most nutritional absorption happens elsewhere in the digestive tract, so the long-term health effects are much less detrimental for colectomy patients than those for people who lose other parts of their GI tract. For some patients the J-pouch is not possible or is ineffective because at the anal connection there remains a small amount of rectum that can still get inflamed. Unfortunately those patients typically end up with an ostomy for life, although many of them find it a welcome relief from the disease.

However, either type of colectomy is typically available only to ulcerative colitis patients. Because their inflammation is restricted to the colon, removing the colon effectively cures their disease. Crohn's disease may likely re-appear elsewhere in the digestive system, so it can not be cured with surgery. Certain complications sometimes require surgery for Crohn's patients, but surgery itself causes scarring in the GI tract which can also be problematic. Therefore surgery is generally avoided with Crohn's except when absolutely necessary.

I'd Give My Appendix for an Outhouse

How my karma became inextricably linked to the bathroom

The same summer when my colitis relapsed and made its chronic nature known to me, I spent several weekends at our family's north-woods Wisconsin cabin. This time I became much more familiar with its bathroom facilities than ever before, visiting them quite often.

It was on one such bathroom break that I realized something interesting. I was sitting in the outhouse we built when I was a kid. I hadn't normally used it much in the summer, but with colitis symptoms, I was running for whatever was closest at the time, so I needed it quite often on that particular trip. While it may be tempting to think that my life first became intertwined with the bathroom as a result of my IBD, some reflection on my past revealed that it really started at a much more formative age. I'm sure I had far more experience with that topic than most kids.

My family spent a lot of time at this lake property while I was growing up. Although we did enjoy a lot of fun activities there, my friends saw it as the place where my parents made us do hard labor. My family preferred to see it as a place to understand the value of hard work and learn to build things. We occupied ourselves building and remodeling, clearing brush, and cutting ski trails through the woods. We typically used the place only in the three warmer seasons, but occasionally we ventured out in the winter for skiing or for some good old weekend hardship.

In northern climates you have to winterize any plumbed house if it will be unoccupied for a significant period—unless of course you want to keep it heated that whole time, which you must do lest the pipes freeze and burst. It's an expensive prospect to replace all the plumbing in that case. To prevent such a disaster you have to empty out all the water lines, drain the water heater, shut down the well, and pour antifreeze down the drains. Reversing this process is a little less complex, but sometimes it's not worth the effort for a couple days of winter wonderland, especially since you have to re-winterize again at the end of your stay.

So, some time during the winter of my junior year in high school, we decided that we needed an outhouse to make winter visits easier by saving us the hassle of these plumbing tasks. We made plans to embark on it the following summer.

As with other projects, this would be another fine example of the *OK Tubesing* approach to construction. *OK* loosely meaning "sufficient" but more accurately and admittedly standing for "Over Kill." When we're not sure if we should use one nail or two, we use three. When we're not sure if we need a 2x4 or 2x6, we use a pair of 2x8s; when we're not sure if our outhouse hole needs to be two or four feet deep, we go six feet down, and for good measure make it six feet square. Overkill? Now that's an understatement, six feet is significantly below the frost line, even in this climate. I guess we like shovels—a lot. A previous year we replaced our septic system drain field ourselves, with shovels. That hole was six feet deep, three feet wide, and twenty-five feet long. And it took a full week to open and close. That was not a fun job, and I wasn't looking forward to undertaking that kind of labor again.

However, now that digging mammoth shit holes was about to become a family tradition, we decided to get bold. This outhouse was going to have enough space for many generations of scat. My sister-in-law is envious. She winters in Fairbanks, Alaska and has no plumbing in her house. (And yes, I mean *winters!* She spends her summers in places you can only get to by sea lion or pterodactyl). In the middle of winter, her outhouse accumulates a dookie spire that piles up because it freezes on impact. It becomes a veritable stalag-shite that needs to be knocked down periodically. Not gonna happen in our super *OK* outhouse.

It became apparent to our collective family consciousness that the biffy needed to be hefty enough to survive a simultaneous earth-quake and tornado attack, so we planned to line the hole with rail-road ties, cross-stacked log cabin style, which would both wall the hole and provide *OK* foundation for the outhouse structure. If need be it could serve as a bomb shelter. It was the eighties after all—the Russians were supposed to be coming at any moment.

One hot afternoon that summer, on a weekend when my mother was out of town, my dad and brother and I started digging. We care-fully peeled off the sod layer on top to replace on a bare spot some-where else in the yard, then started looking for China. Now to make a hole six feet deep and six feet square, you actually have to dig a hole much larger than that, especially in sandy soil that's prone to collapsing. We learned that the hard way on the septic system.

We dug and dug. My dad, famous for point systems and equi-table division techniques for labor and rewards, had come up with a work schedule. We would work twenty-minute shifts, two men on duty and one off at any time. So each person would work forty minutes followed by a twenty-minute break. Perhaps the brilliance of his plan was that we'd get paired up every possible way, provid-ing ample opportunity to relate to each other. It was round-robin father-and-son time. Besides, there was only room for two digging in the hole anyway.

After a few shifts, we were a couple feet down. Maybe three or four even, I'm not sure. On one of my breaks I started getting a stomach ache. It felt like gas pains. I sat on the toilet inside for a while but got no relief. I went back for my shift but was not dig-ging at full strength. The next break I took was extra long. I wanted to wait for that gas to finally leave so I could get back to work. I returned late from this break and left my shift early. It was getting more painful.

At first my dad had his doubts about my situation. Having sloughed off on enough work in the past, I pretty much deserved his skepticism. Plus, it was an ambition of his to teach us what hard work is all about, how to be a good man, to follow through on what you start—the full "Pa Ingalls" values system. And he did a pretty good job of it. So his focus on trying to get me back to work was perfectly reasonable. But after a while something changed his viewpoint. By that time I was on the toilet full time, praying for a fart or two. As my discomfort worsened to more of a stabbing pain in the lower-right abdomen, he started recalling something from his past that I would understand only in hindsight.

Years ago, while recovering from an appendectomy, he had watched a USA Olympic swimming event on TV. While Dad was experiencing such exquisite pain, watching a man pound himself in and out of the water was unfathomable, and the event became etched in his mind. So he had experienced something similar to what I was going through, and suddenly seemed to understand my situation a little better, but I didn't know what he was thinking. I could tell he had an idea, but instead of what parents usually do when you have a simple tummy ache, he made a phone call. I didn't know who he was calling but could hear him on the phone in the kitchen. He talked for a few minutes, then came back and poked me in a few places, asked how it started and how much it hurt (a LOT), and went back to the phone. My folks had several physician friends, and I assumed he had called one of them.

It certainly seemed like my pain was caused by something more than gas. Within the last hour my pain had become excruciating, and by that point I could hardly move. He returned from the phone and asked if I thought I could make it to the car. He explained that he thought I might have appendicitis and that we needed to go into town and get it checked out.

Getting to the car was one thing, but enduring the dirt road and sixty miles of poor pavement back to town was another. I lay on the floor of our van moaning and wincing in pain, agonizing with every bump.

My dad was driving, but not like usual. He is famous for going slow enough to breed tailgaters and resenting them out loud. But not that day. My brother sat in the passenger seat, clearly nervous about my situation, but also excited by something else that was happening. Back then the speed limit was fifty-five. Phil kept peeking at the speedometer and looking back at me. At one point he started using his fingers to communicate our speed. I could tell he was excited, though perhaps he was also trying to offer me refuge from focusing on the pain. He held up seven fingers and mouthed "seventy" silently with wide eyes. My dad, going seventy? Unheard of. He must really be scared. Phil looked back at the dashboard and turned to me again, "seventy-five." I could definitely see excitement this time and wanted to share in it, but I felt like I had a knife in my gut. Plus, if my dad was scared, then I should be terrified.

The rest is sort of a blur. I remember arriving at the emergency room and being poked and prodded by several doctors. Then one came in unbuttoning his lab coat and sat down. He explained that I most likely had appendicitis and that surgery was necessary to be sure and to remove my appendix if it was infected. He assured me that it was a safe procedure but that there were risks, most commonly with anesthesia—one-in-two-thousand chance he said, that surgery and/or anesthesia could be fatal. For the first time in several hours, the gut pain was not at the forefront of my attention. But then he continued, explaining that if it were appendicitis there was at least a fifty percent chance of my appendix rupturing, in which case there was at least a twenty-five percent chance of fatality. Now the surgery didn't sound so bad. While scary either way, the choice was not difficult. [Note that this was more than twenty years ago; I suspect the statistics have improved since then.]

I got a glass of relax-juice of some sort, followed by a blur of surgery prep, some bright lights in a tin room, and a face mask. They asked me a few questions and told me to count backward from ten.

"Ten," and I was out.

I awoke in the recovery room to some commotion. They were moving me around. The nurse made a comment about something "not being good" and started fiddling around with the apparatus attached to me. Down by my feet, the IV bottle was lying on the bed. The tube from my arm was filled with blood which was dissipating into the bottled solution. I suddenly felt very woozy. She picked the IV bottle up and hung it on the post where it belonged. I caught a glimpse of John's face, a chaplain and family friend who years later would become an important mentor to me and eventually officiate at our wedding. I wanted to say hello, but I was too discombobulated to say much, and I drifted out again.

The next three days I spent in a hospital room with another fellow (yep, that was back in the days when surgery called for a sleep-over). He was recovering from some kind of operation too. We agonized together waiting for our gas to come. After surgery they don't let you eat until you start farting because that's a sign that your digestive system has resumed operation. So we sat there hungry and spacey for what seemed like a long time. At one point he had to call the nurse because in his eagerness he got the wrong stuff out.

"I'm terribly sorry miss, but I was trying to push out some bubbles, and I'm afraid I made a mess instead." Poor guy. If only I knew then how some day that very battle would be a major feature of my life.

We both felt fortunate though. The guy in the next room had just been through prostate surgery. He had a grand, deep voice like the tough guy who narrates TV commercials for pickup trucks, but he moaned in rhythm with every breath. Day and night, shaking our walls. He must have been miserable. Occasionally a doctor would come by and ask him to cough; then the rhythmic moans would turn to "No, no, no, no" with every exhale.

"Now Neil, if you don't cough for me we'll have to put the catheter back in."

"No, no. Ow, ow. No, no. Ow, ow..."

At some point, either his meds finally took hold or his pain receded, but eventually we got some peace. Someone had brought me headphones, but I found it difficult to have that much stimulus blaring at me. I was on serious pain killers and getting shots in the butt every few hours, which hurt almost as much as my gut. I lost track of which cheek they'd used last time so just I rolled over to whichever side was more convenient at the time.

It was a painful time, but I had lots of company. My mother had raced back from her trip and was doing double shifts in my room. Something profound in her past, combined with a heroically empathetic soul, gives her superpowers in times like these. My brother stopped by often. At one point he brought a friend along to play Monopoly with me, but I had to make them leave in the middle of the game because they were being so funny I couldn't take the ouchy-laugh any more. I also watched some severe weather through my window with tornado warnings and everything. As my recovery progressed, the nurses made me walk around to prevent pneumonia. There wasn't much to see in my hallway, so I'd shuffle through the double doors to the maternity ward, with IV cart in tow, and watch the newborn babies in their incubators.

By the time I got home, I was feeling pretty good. Actually once I started feeling better I improved quickly. I wasn't allowed to lift anything over ten pounds, but I didn't feel especially bad, so I sat around and watched a lot of movies. Our TV didn't have a remote control, so I couldn't be a total couch potato. But it did seem like I was staying home from school without really being sick—only it was July, so what I was really staying home from was a lot of summer fun, including the outhouse construction.

By the time I got back to the cabin, they had finished digging the hole and had begun to line it with timbers. They were using a sledge hammer to spike the ties together with huge nails about the size of a tent stake, only three times as long. My wimpy ten-pound gimp job was to hand the he-man a new spike and maybe even hold it up to get it started. It was probably a useless job, bordering on interference, but I had to do something, and they were kind to oblige. When our mine shaft was finally complete, they made a Zen garden in the bottom by combing the sand, artistically placing a few choice stones, a leaf, and a piece of driftwood. Whoever christened this crap castle was going to defile something truly beautiful.

We built a roomy six-by-eight-foot structure on top, including windows to allow meditation on the woodsy surroundings and sometimes to watch a deer or porcupine stroll by. The wood we used was salvaged from a garage we dismantled by hand at my grandfather's cabin—his legacy passing down lessons (and fruits) of hard labor to a new generation. We finished it off with a beautiful interior, complete with knotty pine woodwork, wainscoting, and framed art. It's our very own Cistern Chapel. And boy was it built with blood, sweat, and tears—and an appendix.

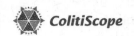

Looking at it now, 20 years later, the OK outhouse is as classy as ever, still struggling to surpass the one-percent fill-line. And it actually survived a tornado that decimated much of the forest nearby. I have no doubt that it will still be there a hundred years from now.

But that outhouse wasn't the cure-all for our scat-management problems. Recently the septic system started making trouble again. Our laborious week-long shovel fest had made it work well for more than two decades, but that's all she had left. Some tree roots made their way up the pipe and into the tank like Neil's urethral catheter. Apparently those trees really liked our contribution to the nitrogen cycle. Plus, the tank was rusting away, so the whole system got replaced. The only painful part this time was watching one guy in a backhoe dig it out, bury a new one, and lay a hundred feet of drain pipe in a single day, without breaking a sweat. Now *that* really hurt.

Nature 9-1-1

As·you envision the urgent potty adventures I keep mentioning, it might help if I let you in on a few more details. Say you're driving down the street and your friend with IBD in the passenger seat asks for a pit stop. This is a secret code. This is your call to duty. You have been enlisted in a mission of epic proportions.

The proper response to this request is never, "Right now?" The answer to that is bloody obvious, literally. What it means is that if you don't get this person to a restroom at the speed of light, your passenger is going to crap his pants in your car. On your leather seats. No air freshener or bobble-headed hula dancer will ever remove that blemish from the psyche of your ride. Then you're going to have to take him home for a shower before your outing can continue. Finding a restroom is a mission-critical objective, and you are the captain. It may be confusing for you. You may not know the best place to look for a bathroom, but trust me, your passenger does. Follow all instructions. Do not pass go, do not collect two hundred dollars, just do what he says. Although he may or may not be fully coherent—let me help you understand.

What's happening in this person's body is not a mere lack of control. It is indeed quite the opposite. This person's ulcerated, bloody, and inflamed colon has been presented with a nasty septic substance full of junk that most people's bodies can store for a while, but his body wants to get rid of immediately. The cells react instinctively, like pulling your hand away from a burning stovetop. This person's colon has assumed control and, without interaction with the brain, is forcing this nasty substance out. The only line of defense this person has is a tiny little sphincter muscle with a hole in it. And it goes to battle with the muscles surrounding the colon. War has been declared. Like a tri-athlete, your friend has been training for this confrontation for years. The battle has been waged a zillion times in a zillion places, and there's no such thing as a draw. There will be a winner and a loser, and it's pretty much 50/50 at best.

There's an intense conversation going on between the brain and the body. You can't hear it but your passenger can. He hears the brain in proper British, and the body in raspy Scottish:

BRAIN: I need full power! Route all auxiliary power to the sphincter.

BODY: Sphincter power at one hundred percent.

BRAIN: Give me maximum power.

BODY: I'm givin' you all she's got, Captain.

BRAIN: Increase reactor power to 120 percent.

BODY: Captain, that could melt down the reactor.

BRAIN: Give me 120 percent, that's an order!

BODY: Reactor at 120 percent Captain; core melt down in ten seconds.

BRAIN: Shut down all unnecessary systems. Route all power to sphincter.

BODY: All systems shut down sir. 120 percent power to sphincter, sir.

BRAIN: Periscope up, look for refuge.

BODY: No power to operate periscope, sir, all power is routed to sphincter.

BRAIN: Give me a ping, we must locate a friendly vessel.

BODY: No power left to ping sir. The sphincter's taken it all. We are blind. And deaf. Five seconds to sphincter failure.

BRAIN: Emergency surface the sub, blow all ballast air.

Like it or not, you're the rescue ship.

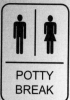

POTTY BREAK

For IBD patients, potty breaks can become an full time occupation. In their households toilet paper must be stocked diligently, bathroom libraries become extensive, and all their "equipment" must function perfectly—and I don't just mean the bathroom fixtures...

A couple summers ago, I dislocated my shoulder in a softball game—for the second time. It happened exactly the same way as the first time—diving back into a base after over-running it. I had vowed never to do that again, but sometimes instinct takes over. Well that was a crippling injury to my wiping arm, which due to my IBD, I desperately needed. Eventually I adapted to using the other one, but it wasn't particularly fun. I guess you never realize how important your wiping arm truly is until you've wiped your ass three hundred times in one day. Managing that task with the wrong hand is no picnic.

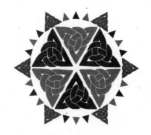

Dr. Spaghetti

After returning home from that summer adventure and relapse, my situation did not improve, despite my work with the newly-found gastroenterologist. I was growing more frustrated with the care I was getting. The original GI specialist my diagnosing surgeon had referred me to was so popular that he was no longer accepting new patients, so I agreed to see another in the same office. I wish I could say good things, but instead I learned a new rule of thumb that one would be wise to hang on to: Never trust a doctor who has an empty schedule. If it's easy to get in, it means everybody else wants to get out. And very soon I did also.

This doctor was sort of like a robot. He could churn out medical terms and explanations in techno-speak, but his softer side was... well...non-existent. While this approach may be effective, or even perfect, for some patients, it wasn't working for me. Minimal in his responses, he was quite mechanical and very difficult to communicate with. He was an emotionless machine, and so I dub him Dr. Tool. I imagine him going home at the end of the day. His wife greets him at the door:

"Hi honey, how was your day?"

"Hi."

She asks him what he wants for dinner.

"Hmmh."

"Isn't there anything you want?"

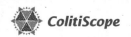

"How about a circular disc of fermented yeast and starch with an exodermal layer of pureed legumes and pasteurized semi-gelatinous lactose."

To which she would (and indeed only she could) reply, "But honey, we had pizza last night."

After another colonoscopy and a year's worth of geologically-layered, rotten consultations as well as unsuccessful fumbling around with Asacol (which never worked for me again), I finally had enough. My symptoms had seen no relief since their first reprise and it was time to find a new advisor. Between the constant aching and half-time occupation on the toilet, I couldn't take it any more. I didn't realize how unnecessary that situation really was until I started talking to other folks who were shocked that I had such severe symptoms for so long without trying something new.

However, without any life-threatening symptoms, I found it very difficult to get treated with priority while attempting to switch to another physician. I called the office and asked to be reassigned. They assured me that it would take several months to get in with someone else, so I would be better off with Dr. Tool. I refused to concur. I insisted. They road-blocked. I called back another day and focused on my acute symptoms, trying for an empathetic response—to no avail. Of course, the phone-answerer wields no power whatsoever except to forward messages—to a scheduler, a nurse, or someone else. Nothing gets accomplished without a callback routine. I got frustrated and gave up.

A couple days later, I called again and talked to a different receptionist who had no idea what I'd spent the last two calls trying to accomplish. I explained again that I was having symptoms and needed some advice, that my current doctor was unsatisfactory and I needed to know if it was worth coming in soon or waiting for a better doctor. As usual she couldn't tell me anything and suggested we send a message to the nurse. I reluctantly agreed and described the problem once more. She read the phone number on file and asked if they could call me at that number. I explained for the umpteenth time that they should remove my work number from their system because I don't want medical calls there, and I provided my cell phone number to replace it. She assured me that a nurse would return my call. I had heard this line many times before. It seemed from my end of the phone that they were running some sort of top-secret operation behind the scenes there.

I envision what is happening at the other end of the call. She writes a message in some unintelligible shorthand on a small sheet of flash paper. She hands it to a messenger standing by who walks it into a neighboring room. It looks right out of a World War II movie—a radio control room with a dozen or so sleepy-eyed operators hunched over desks lined with radio gear. She hands it to one of them who reads it, lights a match, and incinerates the evidence in a momentary flare. He turns to his radio, puts on a pair of head-phones, and starts tapping out code into the key. The signal travels to the nurses' station where an Enigma machine churns out the translation onto ticker tape. The nurse uncurls the strip of paper and reads the message, "Andrew Tubesing, Rectal Hemorrhage, Call at work."

A few hours later, I was at work trying to assemble a delicate electrical circuit at my desk. It was especially frustrating because I'd been interrupted twice already by emergency trips to the restroom. I was building a signal amplifier out of about twenty individual transistors. These circuits are notoriously finicky and seem to stop working if you simply look at them wrong. I tweaked and fidgeted, and finally the signal I was looking for suddenly appeared on the oscilloscope. But it disappeared in a flash. I slightly repositioned my ten fingers, each trying to hold various parts and test probes in position, and the signal returned. Eureka!

The phone on my desk started ringing and posed an interesting predicament. I looked at the phone and back at the amplifier signal on the screen. I couldn't really pick up the receiver, or I'd spoil this precarious success and end up redoing my work a fourth time, so used my elbow to hit the speakerphone button, stretching to reach it.

Just as I answered, "Hello, this is Andy," a couple of students walked into my office seeking help on an upcoming exam. I gave them a look like they were interrupting something, but the message didn't get through. Before I had a chance to stop what was already in motion, the voice on the speaker filled the room,

"Hello, Andrew? This is Melanie from Dr. Tool's office; we got a message that you have rectal bleeding."

There was a moment, frozen, dangling in time, during which nobody in the room could recall a more awkward situation in their life: I was paralyzed, mouth agape. The looks on my students' faces were priceless, as was mine I am sure. The students decided they didn't need help as badly as they had thought and quickly left the room without a word. I lifted a few fingers from my work and the amplifier signal disappeared again. Dropping the scope probes, I picked up the phone receiver to chat with Melanie (I never did get that circuit working again).

"Well yes," I explained, "I think I might need to come in, but I can't bear to see the same guy again. The reason I'm in this situation is because Dr Tool doesn't communicate very well, and I need better information. Maybe I could talk to someone on the phone or come in to see another doctor?

"Mr. Tubesing," she replied, "I can send a message to the scheduler to see if they can get you in with someone else, but it will take a lot longer…"

I probably don't need to reiterate how frustrating this had become. I reluctantly agreed to use the code-talker system once again, hoping for the best but expecting the run-around. When I finally got the call from Captain Logistics, I tried a totally new approach.

"Thanks for your call. I have an urgent situation that has been exacerbated by the incompetence of my current doctor. This phone call is going to end in one of two ways. Either I am going to end up with an appointment for a new doctor within two weeks, or I will be hanging up for good and calling the other GI clinic. Your choice. I have been through the wringer, and this is your last chance."

There was a long pause, followed by some time on hold. I reiterated that Dr. Tool had seen me for the last time. Finally I received an appointment with another gastroenterologist. It was a month away, but I was so happy at the prospect of seeing someone new that I accepted the delay with a smile.

And what a relief it turned out to be for me. The new GI doctor to whom I was assigned finally got my disease under control. With him I was able to establish a problem-solving relationship and have an effective dialogue (not only about IBD but also about politics, which is sometimes a nice diversion). He's a friendly guy, very competent and quite proactive when necessary. Once during a later flare-up that landed me at the Mayo Clinic, he called me at home regularly to check on my progress. For once I truly felt cared for.

He has become my 80 cm Tubemaster. We have these lovely dates every couple months during which we play the gassy Ass-spection video game together. We talk about what we're seeing on screen and the situation with [insert daily politics here]. He has an Italian name that sounds like any of the variety of pasta types whose shapes nobody can correctly identify. He is a welcome and comforting ally in my medical journey, and I couldn't help but name him respectfully after one of my all-time comfort foods. And so it is with affection that I introduce you to Dr. Spaghetti.

*Fear Itself
(is plenty to fear)*

"It's just in your head" is Pure Poppycock

After some introductory appointments to get rolling with the new doctor and make adjustments to my Asacol regimen, we came to a stumbling block for me.

He wanted me to try a new medication that I was very much afraid of—not because of its widely known potential side effects, but rather because I had another very personal reason to fear it.

I had read the volumes of books and web sites that detail each of the IBD medications along with their benefits and drawbacks. Prednisone is what they call a corticosteroid, which is the granddaddy of all anti-inflammatory agents. Not to be confused with anabolic steroids (made famous by unscrupulous athletes), prednisone doesn't have muscle-building effects. It's a completely different kind of steroid, which seriously alters the performance of your immune system by hindering the inflammation process. In my case, we would try to use it to stop my body from generating inflammation in the colon. The theory was that if Asacol couldn't stop the inflammation on its own, we would use prednisone for a short time

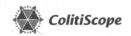

to stop it quickly; then Asacol alone might be able to keep the inflammation at bay.

But some of the side effects of prednisone really freaked me out, though they probably weren't the same ones that concern most people. In order for you to understand my perspective, I need to give you a little background into fear and anxiety issues and how they play into my life.

When Franklin Delano Roosevelt uttered his famous words "The only thing we have to fear is fear itself," I suspect he meant it as an encouraging notion—that our own fear should scare us less than our enemies do. However, in situations where fear itself is the actual enemy, this mantra offers no consolation. Those of us who have experienced crippling fear in our lives know how true his statement is, but not in the way F.D.R. intended.

For those who struggle with anxiety, Roosevelt's words pull out the most fearsome aspect of a situation and use it in an unsuccessful attempt to console us. Imagine if on a transoceanic flight experiencing bad weather and turbulence, the pilot came on the speaker and tried to calm the passengers by telling them that all they have to be afraid of is plummeting out of the sky to a horrible fiery death. Would this make them feel better? Not likely.

For some people, however, anxiety can rear its ugly head without the presence of an actual fearsome event. Some people may read this and wonder why fear should be an issue in cases when there is no immediate physical danger: "It's not a plane crash, it's just fear, so get over it." But for anxious people, fear is indeed the real problem.

Anxiety is a crippling burden which many people bear. It has countless origins and at least as many manifestations—panic attacks being the miserable end game of many such internal battles. The list of potential fear triggers is infinite. Some people fear they're having a heart attack; for some it's post-traumatic stress or a phobic stimulus like heights, closed spaces, dark alleys, etc.; others fear that they can't control things around them. IBD sufferers often develop anxiety because of concerns about their chronic illness and the potential embarrassments faced on a daily basis. For a significant number of people, their anxiety seems to have no tangible origin at all. I have my own set of catalysts—a mixture of IBD issues and other concerns that predated my disease.

Regardless of the source, the basic psychological process is fairly universal for all anxiety sufferers. It begins with a trigger of some kind—perhaps one from the list above, or seemingly nothing at all. This initial catalyst generates the sensation of nervousness or fear. The brain responds, trying to decide how to handle the situation. Generally the person is confused or frightened by what they experience (or what they fear is happening), which magnifies the physical sensations and amplifies the fear signals to the brain. This in turn upgrades the mind's terror alert level. After several of these cycles, the level has ratcheted up, tricking the brain into thinking there is a serious threat. The sufferer starts to worry uncontrollably and begins to feel helpless. Their mind spins out of control with fearful thoughts which lead to catastrophic predictions. Ultimately, they panic.

Once started, this cycle is very difficult to stop. It is also extremely difficult to prevent because after a few rehearsals, this response works like a well-oiled machine, ready to spring to action at the slightest provocation. It is always on "orange alert." In this situation, any sensation associated with fear can set off the chain reaction. Over time the mind learns to associate all fear sensations with the unpleasant panic experiences. Subsequently, the anxious person fears the physical sensations and eventually fear itself.

This can become incredibly invasive because the physiological manifestations of fear are typically the same as those from an adrenaline response, so eventually the brain can't tell the difference between fear and adrenaline, and it responds to both with panic.

The human body reacts to a wide variety of situations with adrenaline. Certainly fear is one of them, but also excitement, joy, arousal, anticipation, thrill, anger, surprise, shock, awe, injury, stress, embarrassment (very common for IBD sufferers!), and just about any significant physio-emotional response. Some of these emotions should be associated with good feelings, some with bad. But for us anxious people, they can all lead to anxiety because of that conditioned response. In addition to feeling anxious during unpleasant situations, we also experience anxiety when we're having intense positive feelings. So as a result, regardless whether

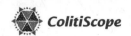

we should be having fun or running for our lives, we face panic—fearing that fear cycle, which has become our generalized response to all adrenaline. And because panic can be the result of both good and bad feelings, all of which are normal, anxiety disorders can have a huge impact on a person's life.

My adrenaline rush starts with a hot forehead and leads to a rapidly pounding heart and shallow breathing. Eventually I develop narrowed peripheral vision and a flurry of fearful thoughts that add fuel to the flames. Instantly or eventually, depending on the situation, it can lead me to outright panic.

This is a classic panic and anxiety situation. I have learned some tools to control the anxiety response process, so nowadays I rarely reach the full panic stage. But it is exhausting. Preventing or stopping the psychological progression from excitement to fear to panic requires an enormous amount of emotional energy.

In fact this struggle can be so challenging that it makes mere physical problems seem like a cakewalk in comparison. The impression that psychological roadblocks should be more easily solved than physical issues because "it's all in your head" is a bunch of hogwash. I've never known a physical problem to be more perplexing and to require more strength and stamina than some of these challenges I've faced in my head.

So, what is it about prednisone that makes it so fearsome for me? Tragically, it causes symptoms just like an extreme adrenaline rush. So the medicine I needed was also likely to provoke my anxiety response to adrenaline, making it an anxiety agent in itself. Isn't that poetic! The medicine with the best chance of helping my physical health is the one with the most potential to challenge my mental health. Talk about adrenaline response, I panicked at the mere thought of it.

As I processed the prospect of taking prednisone I had two reactions. First, I was scared—actually petrified. But second, I was angered by the painful irony of it all. I felt like I was somehow being punished. The anxiety issues were bad enough without the inflammatory bowel disease. But now with the two of them impacting each other in this way, the pain didn't merely add up, instead my misery seemed to be multiplying. How could I deserve this?

I really didn't think I could handle it. Prednisone was the one medicine I hoped never to confront because I was terrified of what it might do to my psychological state. Especially right then. I had my annual summer road trip planned to begin in a couple days. Travel is stressful enough for me; how could I possibly deal with that frightening medication and its effects while I was on the road? I was supposed to attend a high school reunion, visit friends I desperately missed, and do contract work for some old clients (which I needed in order to pay my bills over the summer).

When the doc said we really needed to give prednisone a try, I freaked. It instantly messed up my whole summer plan. I asked for a minute to discuss it with my wife. We chatted, agonized, debated, and lamented. I kept gripping at the space-time continuum trying to be sure this was really happening, looking for a wormhole to elsewhere, anywhere. But I couldn't escape the reality of what I was being asked to confront.

Heather and I came up with a few questions we needed the doctor to answer before we could make a decision. Mostly I wanted to know how long I could wait. I wondered if I could take my trip first and start on the medication after my return. His response to that question changed my life. With just the right amount of elevated emphasis and seriousness in his voice, he said, "What you have to consider, Andy, is that it might make you feel a lot better, and you might have a better trip because of it."

"Really? But I'm leaving in two days, can prednisone really start working that fast?" I had been experimenting with Asacol for a year and a half waiting for it to work, so considering meds with a two-day turn-around was a new concept.

"Yes. This stuff is very powerful; it might start working tomorrow, and you could be feeling a lot better during your trip."

I was stunned. This information suddenly changed all the rules in my head. I started thinking about how wonderful it would be to part with some of my nasty symptoms. I imagined the freedom I might regain—being able to walk to work without worry, make the car trip into the city, stop experiencing such pain and agony...this new possibility changed my outlook instantaneously. I was almost happy, intoxicated for a moment, flying free with the possibility of liberation. Of course, after a few nanoseconds I remembered my fear of the meds, and the fantasy came crashing down in my head, shooting my bird right out of the sky.

Eventually I settled down enough to finish our conversation. I was intrigued but also quite worried. My doctor scribbled a prescription and handed it to me. With great hesitation, I agreed to fill the prescription and do my best to work up the courage to begin to tentatively consider the potential possibility of maybe thinking about perhaps actually taking prednisone. If that sounds a little uncertain, then you got the point. I was very nervous.

We stopped by the pharmacy on our way home, and by the time I got to the house I was already making phone calls—preparing to cancel or postpone my trip. I was really torn up about it. Mostly though, I was too scared to embark upon this new medication experiment with the trip hanging over my head, so I decided to put off the travel part. Sacrifices are a part of life, especially when dealing with a chronic illness. I was terribly disappointed, but considering my other challenges at that moment, I just couldn't deal with a trip.

Now here you have proof of how mental challenges can sometimes be more burdensome than physical ones. Prednisone has a long list of truly harmful physical side effects. The adrenaline rush is one they consider to be innocuous; it's on the list of "annoying" side effects rather than the "dangerous" ones. Here I am, however, with few qualms about the physical damage this medication can cause, yet totally strung out by the so-called silly problem "in my head."

For those who would like to explore the panic and anxiety issue, there is a book I recommend highly. *Hope and Help for Your Nerves* by Dr. Claire Weeks has helped an enormous number of people understand, manage, and overcome their anxiety burden. She has written several other books on the topic as well, any of which is likely to be helpful, but this one worked the best for me.

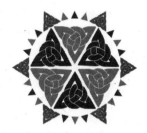

Super-Andy and the Amarillo Miracle

So there I was, having postponed my trip after freaking out about having to start on prednisone, trying to work up the nerve to swallow the little orange pills. I started thinking out loud.

"They look like overgrown baby aspirin, but they hardly give me the comforting feeling I remember from childhood. Actually they're not really orange, they're more of a salmon color. They're chalky. They look like they won't go down very smoothly. Do we have any pudding? I should really take these with pudding. Chocolate would be nice; I like chocolate. Mmmmm chocolate," I concluded sounding like Homer Simpson.

"Are you just stalling?" Heather asked.

"Yeah, probably," I replied.

"That's my Andy," she said with a charmed tone and a knowing look in her eye. She revels in identifying those situations when I'd rather bury my head in the sand than follow through with something fearsome. I freely admit to an occasional streak of denial; though it's rarely fun to be called on it. But she has a way of making that benevolent condescension somehow sound like a warm fuzzy.

Her efforts to console me were appreciated, but they were not working. I was pretty nervous. I felt the same trepidation that comes

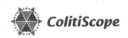

with the clickety-clack sound of a roller coaster ratcheting its way up the first incline, preparing to launch me into the fearsome unknown. I shivered at the thought—I don't even have to be on the ride for that sound to disturb me. The anticipation alone is torturous. I took a deep breath.

"I guess I really don't have a choice. I've been miserable for over a year, and obviously the Asacol isn't going to work again," I said.

"The doctor said prednisone might really work, so don't you think it's worth a try? It might be awful, or it might not, but we both know that if you don't take it you're guaranteed to be miserable," Heather reasoned.

"Yeah," I sighed, and took another deep breath. This one came out sputtered because I was trembling slightly. I could see my reflection upside-down in the surface of the water as I looked into the glass tumbler in front of me. I peered through the water at the pills in my hand; they looked comically enlarged and distorted. I was distracting myself again.

I am really not a pill-popper. I don't even take Tylenol unless I really need it. When I dislocated my shoulder, I didn't take the pain meds they prescribed. When my back seized up in spasms for a week, I couldn't bring myself to use the muscle relaxants they gave me; though that probably wouldn't have mattered anyway since everybody except the doctors has figured out they're useless on back pain.

"What does it say they'll do again?" I asked. Heather picked up the pharmacy fact sheet and started reading off the side effects. "Never mind, I don't want to hear it," I quickly decided.

"Sweetie," she said, taking my hand from across the table and leaning into me. "I won't let anything bad happen to you."

I thought for a moment.

"OK then," I said with a sudden, mostly fake, air of confidence, "Here goes."

I popped two tablets into my mouth and took a couple swigs of water. The pills were so dry and chalky that they stuck to my tongue and sort of skidded toward the back of my mouth. A foul taste circulated. They definitely didn't taste like baby aspirin. I took a couple more swallows, and the pills reluctantly made the turn down my esophagus, leaving streaks of pasty bitterness on my taste buds.

"We should have made pudding," I remarked, disguising my discomfort—mostly from myself. Heather chuckled and looked me in the eye. It was a comforting look and it settled me down a little.

This is the part I hate the most. Doing something like that and then waiting for it to take effect. I was hyper-aware of every sensation, worried about everything, hoping to keep my composure, nearly failing more than once. I did my best to distract myself, keeping busy around the house for a while.

I don't have a lot of specific memories from the remainder of that afternoon and night, aside from a general impression of what it was like to be on the prednisone. Yeah, it was an adrenaline high for sure, and it came with other physical effects too. My cheeks were tingly, and I was sweating profusely. Overnight my shirt would get soaked in my sleep, and I'd have to get up and change.

Over the next couple days, the medication was clearly affecting me. I could tell that I was more agitated. I was interacting with things (and Heather) more intensely. She said it seemed like I was vibrating—buzzing with energy. I jumped from task to task and thought to thought with punctuated haste. It really was like being high on adrenaline. Under these circumstances, luckily, it was fairly easy to keep busy. I cleaned off my desk, caught up with some filing, and did a bunch of tidying-up I would never usually spend time on. The jitters got so intense at times that Heather would laugh and say, "You're doing it again, you're getting twitchy."

I didn't always notice, which is more to say that I managed to forget about it occasionally, perhaps out of necessity. But she could not help but notice.

"It's like you're Super Andy, running around and overdoing everything." She said. The blue suit and red cape came to mind immediately. I beat my chest and felt for a moment like Tom Hanks when he finally made fire in *Castaway*. It wouldn't surprise me if a person felt the urge to fly in my situation. I wasn't delusional, just really hyper. My uncle, who had also experienced prednisone, gingerly described it as "feeling jazzed up." That's a subtle way to describe an experience that felt about as subtle as a sledgehammer

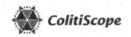

to me at the time. I did understand, however, that it was normal to be experiencing these sensations under such circumstances.

Up to this point my colitis symptoms were quite predictable, as in "bad all the time." I had bloody mucous number-twos about every twenty minutes. I couldn't pass gas except on the toilet because it was never dry. Tenesmus gave me dry heaves out the rear end every time I sat on the toilet. Any time there was stool passing through, it came out in painful bursts—this time like passing a pinecone *against* the grain. My rectum ached. Not a sharp or specific pain, just a solid, residual ache somewhere between my tailbone and perineum—as if it were bruised somehow. It was impossible to relieve. I had been feeling this way for about a year and a half.

The thought of making a two-day road trip for a six-week stay up north was unimaginable. I had fantasies of renting an RV to make the journey so I could just sit on the toilet the whole time. But if I did that, somebody else would have to drive, and Heather needed to stay home for some training. She planned to meet me up there later in the summer. So if I went, I would have to go alone. With such burdens on my mind, I canceled the trip. I felt that I had no choice. At the time, I thought that even if my symptoms miraculously improved, I would be too uncomfortable about being on prednisone to take a trip. So I let it go. I canceled my reunion reservation and bowed out of the golf tournament. I called my clients and advised them that I had been delayed indefinitely due to health concerns and would need to reschedule the contracting work.

Then I settled in for what could be best described as an uncharted holding pattern. This is very unusual for me. During the summer, I typically know exactly how I need to spend my time to make the schedule work out, and the logistics often get complicated. Clearing my schedule and keeping it open so I could go with the flow felt pretty unnatural.

So there I was hanging around the house, climbing the walls, looking for tall buildings to leap in a single bound. Heather was generally amused by it all but found me a bit overwhelming at times. I felt pumped up most of the time. I tackled tasks with remarkable enthusiasm, but the kind that sometimes brings hasty, regrettable results. I didn't cut off my finger with a table saw or anything, but

I'm pretty sure I wasn't operating very carefully or efficiently. I did stay off the motorcycle though—that was definitely a good idea.

Luckily, I managed to not let anxiety get the better of me (for the most part), though it was a challenge.

Sometimes I get a glimpse of the survival mode my subconscious goes into when it knows I need protection. Sort of like the dream I had while getting my wisdom teeth pulled—I was browsing around the outside of an oppressive wall that leaned out over me. I was killing time, somehow aware that there was heartache on the other side and that I was having that dream for the express purpose of covering over an otherwise traumatic event, protecting myself from it. That was a powerful experience for me; it gave me confidence that if push came to shove, my brain might be able to pull out the stops and save me from myself. It's comforting to remember that.

The fact that I had something tangible to blame my craziness on did make the whole experience easier for me. Contrary to what I feared, for the most part I was able to compartmentalize the unpleasant feelings as direct effects of the steroids. Plus the prednisone brought some other less familiar symptoms, so it was different enough from my normal anxiety triggers to be distinguishable. Instead of constantly wondering and worrying about all the fearsome sensations and behaviors, I could simply chalk it up to prednisone and carry on with other thoughts. It gave my mind a rocket boost to reach escape velocity from the anxiety cycle, breaking my orbit around the black hole of panic. It was tough at times for sure, but that little bit of self-protection went a long way toward keeping me sane during that time. And it still works. More than four years later I continue to endure the same battles. I still hate it when I get the crazies, but I have learned to live with it.

After a couple days I actually was getting symptomatic relief. The doc said that prednisone could work powerfully and quickly, but I really was skeptical after such a long, unsuccessful experience with Asacol. Thankfully, he was right. The aching disappeared. The frequency of bowel movements reduced exponentially. Even the evidence of blood seemed to taper off. I was beginning to understand his insistence on having me try it. And I was glad I had the courage to follow through. It was like coming out of the dark, a

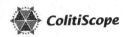

burden being lifted. I adapted fairly quickly to my rising freedom. I walked to campus for the first time in many months. I ate food without running to the bathroom immediately. I slept the whole night without ass-piss. I went to the driving range.

Rediscovering these luxuries started to change my outlook. I got to thinking that maybe I could take the trip after all. It was too late for me to arrive in time for the reunion, but I could still make it to start my work projects on schedule. Heather and I talked about it, making a list of potential problems and solutions. If things got bad, I could stop in a hotel or come home if need be. I had friends along the way in St. Louis, so that felt like a possible refuge. Perhaps I should bring a bucket along in the truck. It started to look like I could actually travel. So I started planning again; if symptoms were still improving the next day I might actually go.

After another night of uninterrupted sleep, the first of three miracles occurred. I got up in the morning, and I peed standing up! For the first time in more than a year I had to go number one worse than number two. I stood there marveling, rediscovering that characteristic activity only boys get to do—and take for granted until a moment like this. Sheer elation. Even better, a while later I had my first solid poop in at least eighteen months. The clouds parted and light shone down from the heavens; angels sang in chorus; the planets aligned. Heaven on Earth. Miracle number two, literally.

I called my friend Chris to tell him about the experience. I was all excited; his enthusiasm may have been tempered by the fact that I woke him up, but being familiar with the misery I'd been enduring, he seemed to understand the greater meaning of my news.

"Cool dude," he croaked in a groggy voice. I let him go back to sleep.

I started packing. My work equipment lived in the truck, so it didn't take long to load up the other supplies, already organized in totes in my own tidy way. I filled a bag and a laundry basket with clothes and loaded my briefcase with the files and records I needed. I even put together some snacks for the road, should I be daring enough to eat in the car. This trip was really going to happen. I made one last check for essential cargo, and I hit the road, three days late, but early enough to still fit in most of the activities I had planned.

I headed east toward Texas. There's a whole lot of nothing along that stretch of road, and if I needed a bathroom, I wouldn't be likely to find one. The nice thing was that I did pack the bucket and a couple rolls of TP for the road, and on the desolate landscape, a makeshift nature-biffy wouldn't be too hard to muster up, though finding some privacy might be a challenge.

I got daring, eating some crackers and drinking a bottle of water. So far so good. Actually I was stunned by how easy it is to eat when you don't have to be afraid of what it will do to you. Since the previous morning, I hadn't experienced a single emergency BM, and my situation seemed only to be getting better.

About midafternoon I hit Amarillo and got off the freeway for a break. I needed to find a wide-brimmed hat so I could avoid getting sunburned on the golf course, assuming I'd soon be regaining the freedom to play a few holes. I drove around a bit and found a Shepler's western wear store a few blocks off the interstate. It was a huge building that resembled a wild-west horse barn, with vaulted ceilings and exposed wooden beams. For once I didn't have to head straight for the bathroom when I got out of the car. Wow, what a luxury.

I shopped around and found the perfect cowboy hat. But actually I make that sound simpler than it was. I didn't shop so much as obsess, as usual—accessorizing is important business. Not only did I have to consider every hat in the store, but once I picked the style I wanted, I tried on the whole stack of my size to find the perfect fit. The one I selected was sort of pre-ragged and soft, so it didn't look like formal rodeo dress-up but more casual country-boy. It reminded me of Brad Pitt and his hat in *Thelma & Louise,* but I knew better than to think anyone would confuse the two of us in the slightest. I had the blonde drawl-talking cutie at the service desk install a few ventilation rivets in it for me, but I wasn't brave enough to tell her I planned to use it for golf. I'm pretty sure that's sacrilegious in some way—driving cattle and driving golf balls aren't really in the same league…at least not in Texas.

I paid for my new golf/rustling outfit and headed outside. It was hot. The filling in the asphalt cracks was oozing. *It's barely June,* I thought to myself, *I'm sure glad I don't live here.* Then it began to emerge, miracle number three started its gradual magic.

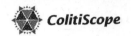

I looked across the parking lot and saw my truck, and behind it rising up into the sky like a bright shining beacon was a Wienerschnitzel sign. Ohhh man, I hadn't eaten a chili dog in many months. Without thinking I was already driving straight toward it. A creepy voice in my head echoed "Precious, my precious…"

Somehow, through the remarkable, confidence-building events of the last twenty-four hours, my mindset had been completely transformed. A day earlier I would not have even noticed that sign—I had become so accustomed to tuning out fast food, especially while out driving around, that I would never have eaten in the car. Now suddenly I was in the drive-thru line at Weinerschnitzel ordering lunch. And here it comes, the grand finale. Drum roll please…I left the drive-thru window, got right back on the interstate, and ate two chili dogs ON THE ROAD!

Sweet mercy.

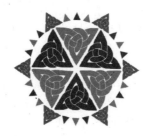

Kryptonite

Yes prednisone solved a lot of problems. Good things happened. The summer trip up north went pretty well. My symptoms became quite manageable, and I regained many freedoms I had come to miss. Life was much closer to normal than it had been for a long time.

It wasn't all easy though. In fact, I would never get over the steroid factor fully. I am still adapting to the crazy mood swings as they come and go, so it is still stressful, even to this day. The jazzed up super-Andy sometimes does fine on prednisone, but sometimes it drives me nuts.

Prednisone replaces a job your adrenal glands normally perform. It metabolizes into prednisolone, which is similar to chemicals produced by the adrenal glands. It's natural in your body at levels of around five milligrams per day and is doled out by the endocrine system to control lots of internal functions, including adrenaline responses and the inflammation process. When you're taking a daily dose of prednisone that exceeds your body's normal level of prednisolone, it is overabundant in your system all the time. As a result, the adrenal glands shut down because they don't need to produce their own hormones with all those steroids in your system already. This is why it's important to not stop taking prednisone suddenly. Instead the dosage must be tapered down to zero slowly, to allow time for the adrenal system to start doing its job again.

On a high enough daily dose, the levels are sustained in my body, so there's no change in the adrenaline-like sensations. I think in that case my brain filters it out and I am able to ignore it for the most part. However, while taking an intermittent dosage like the every-other-day schedule I am on now, the adrenal system is constantly starting up and shutting down, which results in sporadic levels of prednisone in my system. It is also troublesome when the dosage is changing or has changed recently. Unfortunately this is a significant strain on my mind. The fluctuations cause spikes in my adrenaline level, and it's impossible to not notice.

[The calculus nerds in my audience might be intrigued by my initial description of this process, which I re-wrote for the benefit of general readers. Originally I proposed that the steroid level in my bloodstream is defined by the $f(x)$ function, and the fluctuating level represents the function's derivative, which is the rate of change of the prednisone level. I am happiest when the derivative is zero, meaning a stable drug level. I start to get uncomfortable with any non-zero derivative, which corresponds to a fluctuating level. I become outright miserable with steeply sloped derivative values (especially when they approach the impulse function, which happens with an infinite derivative or vertical slope) as is common on the two-day "binary" dosing cycle.]

I don't always find it problematic, but it can be quite annoying. Keeping the anxiety machine in check with all those peaks and crashes can be very stressful. Even when I'm not feeling the sensations, I know I've taken the meds. Often I'm on edge, just waiting for the rush to come. This anticipation can be just as disconcerting as the real thing.

One approach that helped to some extent was to determine the best time of day to take the medicine, which required some experimentation. The later in the day I took it, the harder it was to sleep at night. Oh the other hand, I couldn't bring myself to have it for breakfast either. I finally settled on midmorning, which allowed me time to wake up and adjust to the day before stirring things up. I also found it easier to be experiencing the peak of the side effects while I was busy during the day. With distractions I was less likely to fixate on the unpleasant sensations.

While the prednisone gives me super powers to suppress the inflammation in my colon, it works like kryptonite on my nerves, weakening my defenses while it's in my system. And that's a battle I have to keep fighting, at least for now.

The one consolation in all of this is that I now have an identifiable source to blame the jitters on. Before I was taking medications that could induce the anxiety symptoms in my body chemistry, I would always jump to panic trying to figure out where my anxiety sensations came from. *What is causing them? Would I be able to endure them? Would they traumatize me? Would they ruin the panic-free momentum I've built up over the last few days/weeks/months, etc.?* Of course those feelings and questions naturally create fear themselves and thus restart the vicious cycle. But now that there's a physiological reason for my body to be experiencing adrenaline peaks, I can sometimes blame the sensations on the prednisone, and carry on with minimal interruption.

I say "sometimes" because it doesn't always work. Today for example, I was having trouble with my prednisone. It's an "on" day which means by the time I took my meds this morning it had been forty-eight hours since my previous dose. A few hours later I started getting the tell-tale tingles in my cheeks. My forehead got hot. My vision became affected. I am facing that ever-familiar mental battle to keep calm. It's hard to stay relaxed. Sometimes a nap is nice because sleep can reset my thought processes—if I am lucky enough to fall asleep under such conditions.

Usually when I start feeling this way, I need a distraction—something else I can focus on to divert my energy elsewhere. Today I decided to write about it as I had promised myself I would do when I was experiencing my disease intensely. While it's not exactly a distraction, it was a new approach to this particular situation.

The trouble is that writing about this topic is inherently the opposite of what I feel I need at the moment. I want to forget about this particular symptom, and not focus on it because dwelling on it is precisely what makes my anxiety worse. But today I am courageously trying the writing approach. Partly for your benefit, but also to see if perhaps it might serve as a distraction after all. Actually it has worked. After typing for a couple hours, I feel much better.

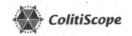

Perhaps now I should get on with what I was really supposed to do this afternoon. Not that I'm trying to skirt the issue, but the trouble with *exploring* my anger and fear is that, in the process, I inevitably *experience* anger and fear. That's why it's always nice to keep a dose of denial handy, and on that note I think I'll shift focus.

It is quite normal for IBD patients to experience a high level of fear and stress. There's a lot to worry about while living with this disease. Clearly I have an anxiety source that originated in my life long before the colitis arrived. But, as an IBD patient myself, I often experience many of the classic IBD-generated triggers as well.

It's interesting to look back on the times when I was quite sick, before I was able to control my colitis with medication. I was running to the bathroom all the time. My wife was working 80 miles from home and spent weeknights at an apartment there. I was driving back and forth a lot, and this was a long trip across a desert with up to thirty miles between bathroom facilities. I was lecturing and teaching long lab sessions during which it would be difficult to sprint for the restroom—all while having extremely urgent bathroom needs, sporadic bouts of extreme discomfort and pain, and constant worry about the impending humiliation I might experience at any moment. Even now, when I feel healthy most of the time, these concerns still surface quite often.

This kind of life would provoke anxiety in any person. As a result, many IBD patients develop anxiety issues—even if they didn't have anxious nerves before the onset of digestive illness. So I sometimes wonder how I survive those bouts of uncertainty and worry, especially with my extra layer of fear triggers. But then I remind myself that the worst thing I have to be afraid of IS fear. The other challenges are not fear itself, they are tangible events and therefore they have practical, effective solutions. That understanding is critical in helping me get through the unpleasant times.

Over time, the physical burdens of inflammatory bowel disease did start to affect my stress level. I didn't notice it so much while it was happening because each additional obstacle was adding a thin, but somewhat opaque, layer to my emotional state. No individual challenge on my list was so fearsome on its own. But if you stack up enough vellum, eventually light will stop getting through. Over months and months of layering, progressively my stress level had become quite thick and heavy. Sometimes it was hard for me to see much light through it all.

When I first started on prednisone my symptoms improved over a matter of days. As many of the stress-inducing complexities of my life dissolved away, I developed an emergent sense of freedom— literally like an uncaged bird. Only then did I realize how much my anxiety level had crept up over time. Sure I had been aware of the obvious ways in which my life was stressful. But here I was, an expert on my own anxiety, yet still shocked by the insidious nature of stress building up without my awareness.

So, while prednisone gave me the Super-Andy power to live more comfortably in terms of physical symptoms and practical day-to-day worries, it also worked like kryptonite—challenging my anxiety cycle in other ways. Every superhero has a weakness after all.

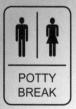

POTTY BREAK

Since we mentioned the effects of stress buildup in this chapter, I thought I'd relate this story. To me it illustrates how the brain doesn't always function properly while processing anxiety.

We were flying into Albuquerque one night during a thunderstorm. Landings there are often rough because of the windy desert and the mountains surrounding the airport. It was really rocky and bumpy. The plane was tilting back and forth and bouncing all over the place. I had to use the bathroom really badly, but the seatbelt sign was on, and I didn't want to face-plant myself into the ceiling, so I had to wait.

Fortunately we were in the front of the plane, so as soon as it stopped at the gate I leaped up to be the first one out. I blazed up the jetway and into the gate area, immediately spotting a pair of bathrooms across the hall. I sped inside and got seated in a heartbeat. Just as things started flowing, I realized something strange. I was hearing a clip-clop sound. Not the kind made by wing-tips and work boots either. No, these sounded like narrow heels.

I wondered to myself, *Do you hear any male voices? No. Did you see any urinals on the way in? No.* I leaned forward to peek out just as I heard a female dialogue enter from the hallway and pass my stall door. *OOPS!*

I finished quickly and exited with my face in my hands, looking down at the floor and hoping nobody would notice. *Phew!*

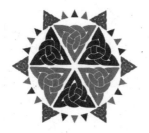

Bus-ted

That summer road trip up north after my introduction to prednisone reminded me of another bathroom connection in my past. Driving has always been one of my favorite activities. I can entertain myself for ungodly periods of time without music or conversation. Long or short trips, going anywhere is fine with me, I love being on the road. It soothes me. It's my meditation time. It's when I feel alive. So it shouldn't surprise you that I've found it harder to get my spiritual reflection time on the road while I've had the symptomatic complications of IBD. Driving is a lot less fun when you're afraid to stray more than ten seconds from the can. But I do get relief often enough to venture out and find my peace, and this cross-country trip came with welcomed ease after what I'd been through the previous eighteen months.

I have a particular penchant for large vehicles and have driven everything from motorcycles to eighteen-wheelers. I enjoy the challenge of operating a complex machine, the spatial intuition of maneuvering, and the geographic adventure of being on the road. So, in the previous decade when I had a chance to drive a school bus in Duluth during a time between jobs, I jumped at the opportunity. Why not add another vehicle to my repertoire?

I got more than I bargained for, however. There was so much more to that job than driving. Babysitting seventy screaming kids while trying not to run them off the road is not exactly the kind of

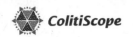

on-the-road meditation I normally find relaxing. It's a tricky job because you're completely responsible for this precious cargo but have absolutely no power or authority to control it.

My afternoon bus route started at an elementary school about halfway up a steep urban slope much like those in San Francisco. Houses and buildings were all carved into the hillside at dramatic angles. I would take the kids down the hill, through downtown, and out onto the narrow sand bar which divides the harbor from the open water of Lake Superior. There's a single street running its six-mile length with beach homes on both sides. I would drive out to the end, dropping the kids on the south side of the street, and back in dropping them on the north side. When I finished that route, I headed back through downtown and up to the hilltop to pick up a load of high school kids, taking them in a different direction.

One day, while bringing my first load of kids down the hill, my bus started smoking from the rear. Badly. There was a great plume developing behind me, and the air inside was starting to get opaque and reeked with the smell of burning material. There was no place to pull over, so I had to stop in the street. I took a quick look in my interior mirror to see every single one of the seventy faces, bodies straining against the railing behind me, all looking like they were scared for their lives. It didn't smell like fire exactly but more like smoke made by super-heated materials or scalding oil. It was coming from the rear of the bus where there's no engine or flammable components. I picked up the radio and called in to my company's dispatcher. I was bus number 218.

ME: Two-eighteen to base.

DISPATCH: Go ahead two-eighteen.

ME: I have a severely smoking bus.

DISPATCH: Is it a fire, two-eighteen?

ME: Negative. At least I don't think so; it's coming from the back.

DISPATCH: What's your location?

ME: Just heading down the big hill through downtown.

long pause

> DISPATCH: Two-eighteen, is your parking brake on?
> *longer pause*
> ME: Two-eighteen is under way. Over and out.

Yeah. That little exchange was broadcast to the entire fleet of a hundred buses. I could virtually hear the collective laughter of all those drivers spread across town. I took a LOT of ribbing for that one, in fact there was a sizeable group of drivers waiting for me at the terminal when I returned. They had stayed around before going home, waiting to give me a round of applause when I walked in the door with my paperwork.

Looking back on that experience reminded me of another story that suggests the bathroom challenge wasn't a totally new thing for me. Before the days of my diagnosis, I did have some abnormal digestive issues; though at the time I don't think I realized they were unusual. I'm pretty sure I had colitis for a long time before it ever became acute enough to cause concern. There were definitely times when I needed a bathroom quick. I called them EPs (emergency poops), or sometimes RNP (right now poop), or for extreme cases, RFNP (you get the idea).

There weren't a lot of opportunities to make a pit stop on my school bus route—it was dense urban territory, rarely offering a place to park a school bus or to find a public restroom. Besides, I couldn't leave students on the bus unattended, so I really had no options when there were kids on board. There was, however, one lone retreat—a fast food joint in the little tourist area wedged between downtown and the sand bar. After I dropped the last of the early load, if I had time before the high school pick-up, I would occasionally stop there midway. There was a nice big shoulder where I could park the bus while I went inside for a snack or a smoke and a potty break if needed.

One of those times I approached this personal rest stop in a bit of a hurry. I had needed a bathroom break since midroute but had no way to stop. It was getting quite urgent, but as long as I stayed seated I thought I could contain it. I quickly parked my bus on the shoulder and sprinted inside to do my business. I wasn't gone for a terribly long time, maybe five or six minutes, but when I came out I noticed quite a traffic problem developing in the street.

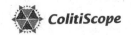

It seemed that there was logjam of some sort; a long line of stopped cars was trailing behind my parked bus. I spent a moment pondering this occurrence because I could see up the street and there was no congestion there. Then it suddenly hit me. I had forgotten to turn off the lighting system, so when I opened the door to get out of the bus, it turned on the flashing red lights and extended the stop arm, bringing traffic to a halt. I was in such a hurry to get inside that I didn't notice, and my bus had been holding up traffic the whole time.

I ran for the bus, clambered inside quickly, and shut off the lights. I felt stupid enough that I hid under the dashboard until all the cars had passed. What a testament to courteous Minnesota drivers though; making that mistake in certain other places would have generated mayhem, I'm sure.

Years later I was telling these stories to some in-laws at a family gathering. They laughed a lot at the first story. They howled at the second. Then one of Heather's cousins said something that got the most laughter of all,

"So Andy, I'm starting to get a picture of why you *used to be* a school bus driver."

Touché!

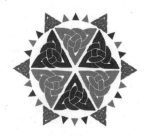

Bionic Bunghole

Although the prednisone does a pretty good job of controlling the inflammation and keeping my symptoms at bay, I noticed that they ebb and flow over time. Minor flares and ill-advised menu choices have caused unexpected urgencies, even when I've seemed to be pretty healthy. I was back home after my summer travels. The school year was underway, and I started experiencing one of those 'flow' periods, if you know what I mean. It's such a familiar story to me now, I can envision it vividly. Here's the way it went.

As I did so many times a day, I leapt up from my desk and scrambled for the door. My quintessential decision—left turn or right turn? To the left was a more private bathroom in the back hallway, and it was closer—but only if the workshop was open for a shortcut. To the right was the public restroom, slightly farther and much less private, but it was a straight path. I looked at my watch, 11:55…hmm was the shop still open or would I have to go outside to get to the back hallway? A dangerous detour, too close to lunch time I decided, better not chance it.

I turned right and started speed-waddling down the hall toward the public restroom. My mind was in a turmoil. Would this be the day of my consummate humiliation? My heart raced as I realized that class started in 40 minutes—barely enough time to run home for a shower if the unthinkable happened. But I wouldn't finish my grading in that case, and the students would not be happy. As

I started to panic, the rectal pressure tried to overwhelm me. It would take a determined mind to go the distance. I felt it straining to get out—Old Faithful unnaturally delayed from its rigid geological destiny. Did I have the power, the stamina, the sheer will to alter the course of planetary geology? Maybe so, god I hoped so…maybe not. Arrgh no, focus! Focus! I shuffled faster, passing some students going the other way.

They gave me a funny look. I wondered if they could hear the "Bionic Man sound" that I was hearing. *Nak nak nak nak nak. Nak nak nak nak nak.* "We have the technology, we can rebuild him…" These students might not have even known what that sound was. After all they were young enough to think Michael Jackson was always white. Actually, they probably thought Steve Austin was a pro wrestler. How pathetic. Stone Cold Steve Austin couldn't stand a chance against Six Million Dollar Steve Austin. No way. Plus, there's no way Stoney-boy could ever take on Bigfoot. Not a chance. Only the Six Million Dollar wonder could defeat Sasquatch in a two-part season finale.

Those poor 20 year-olds were being misled so. They'd never know that strange sound they heard was a miracle of modern man (or at least a 70's version). They'd live the rest of their lives never knowing they'd borne witness to the Bionic Bunghole.

Nak nak nak nak nak. Nak nak nak nak nak. I heard it loudly; I needed to hear it. It was my mantra, my backbone. I was determined. I focused on the corner approaching, which I turned sharply, grazing it. I slalomed back to the left for the final approach, arm extended. I burst through the door, and it was an outright scramble. My right hand automatically unbuckled my belt; my left arm grabbed at the stall door, closing, and latching it in one swift rehearsed motion. *Nak nak nak nak nak,* louder now; both hands thrust at the waist of my pants as I lunged backward and hit the seat flying at a 45 degree angle, skidding to a halt on the cold surface with a chirp. *Waaahhahahahhaha!* My brain let out such a relief I could hardly hear my own thoughts as my body shuddered in both ecstatic relief and severe pain. Did I make that sound out loud? I wasn't even sure. I didn't care—I made it!

"We are the champions…we are the champions…" the bionic sound in my head had given way to the celebratory words of Queen,

complete with chorus and wailing guitar. I had prevailed. The Bionic Bunghole, pumped up and toned by six million events just like this one, had again saved the day. But in the TV show they surely would have cut to commercial before all the pain started. Cramping and heaving, I made a lot of sounds unbecoming of either Steve Austin, but hey, I haven't actually been rebuilt, I only got one quasi-bionic part.

My private victory party was cut short by the sound of someone entering the bathroom. I was pretty much done by then, slumped back, spent and limp. My arms sprawled over the handrails. Knees and ankles twisted strangely, I breathed a special breed of exhaustion. The hoarse feeling in my throat reminded me I had not suffered quietly.

I eventually finished the paperwork and headed back to my office, fatigued and relieved—and no one was the wiser to it. Too bad it was an anonymous achievement though, because this athletic feat, this milestone of human strength and determination, deserved a trophy. Or a medal at least. On Colonel Bunghole's dress uniform there should be a vast array of those little ribbon-metals stacked together on the breast—and the jump suit plastered with mission patches, to signify triumph over countless such endurance tests. It's a new breed of heroics.

Yep, even when I'm feeling pretty good, the ebb can suddenly turn to flow, sometimes for no apparent reason, and I must immediately leap right back into the same heroic action drama once again.

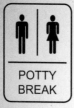

POTTY BREAK

On one similar occasion I did not make out so well—I had a disaster in fact, and there was only a very short time before class started. I did my best to recover but truly needed to go home to finish the job (luckily I still lived in town at the time). Sitting on a plastic bag in the car, racing home, I was stopped by a campus cop. It was really not fun at all.

"Late for class or something?" he asked.

"Um, yeah. Something like that."

I got off with a warning, which I think is the only time in my life I didn't get a ticket when stopped for speeding. Maybe the officer realized I had bigger problems. I guess if I were ever going to get such a break, that was the perfect time for it.

Downward Spiral

Over that school year, my gastroenterologist and I did a fair amount of experimentation, trying to find other effective medications to replace the prednisone, which we intended to use for only a short time to suppress the acute inflammation. I was still on Asacol at maximum dosage, and our attempts for it to work on its own without prednisone had failed. So we added another drug called azathioprine which is an immunomodulator (also known by the brand name Imuran). Similar to 6-Mercaptopurine (6-MP), this drug suppresses the immune system in a different way than prednisone.

The azathioprine side effects are much less common than the nearly inevitable problems prednisone can cause. We were hoping that it could take the place of prednisone (and possibly the Asacol too) for a long-term solution.

As we had done with Asacol, we tried increasing doses incrementally, each time slowly lowering my prednisone dosage as far as possible, attempting to determine if the azathioprine would work on its own. Unfortunately, each time the prednisone got below a certain level my symptoms would begin to return.

The maximum safe azathioprine dosage is determined experimentally for each patient with blood tests that monitor its toxic components in the body. Once I reached my maximum we tried again to back off the prednisone to no avail. At this point it seemed

like I might be looking at prednisone for a longer term than originally expected, unless we could find something else to take its
place.

During this time my system was fairly stable, other than the
short spurts of symptoms that came with minimal prednisone doses. But it all changed that spring, nearly a year since I had started
on the steroids.

People say that IBD can flare up during stressful times. I am
fairly certain that's true for me. I've noticed that symptoms sometimes worsen during the burden of travel, the semester-end crunch
time, and the holidays. That particular spring turned out to be full
of unusual catalysts to restimulate my symptoms. The first in this
chain of stressful events was the death of my last living grandparent.
That was directly followed by the suicide of a colleague, then two
more deaths—a family friend and another more distant relative. All
of these events occurred within a week of each other. While the first
two hit much closer to home, the onslaught of morbidity brought on
by the second two certainly multiplied the impact on me. My folks
had several other funerals to attend during that time as well, and
collectively we felt bombarded by this message that life is awfully
fragile. Adding to that, Heather and I were in the midst of selling
our house and making home shopping trips to the city every weekend. I am sure you can imagine that we had a lot on our minds.

My health started deteriorating. I had been getting symptomatic indications that things were going downhill. Mucus was back;
cramping and tenesmus were showing up now and then. To complicate matters, I had been trying to taper down the prednisone, which
was likely contributing to my worsening symptoms as well.

I was supposed to make a birthday trip to Las Vegas with my
wife and brother, but my health was not cooperating. I ended up
canceling that trip, which turned out to be especially disappointing
because Heather had secretly arranged for my cousin and his wife
to meet us there as a surprise. They were going to stroll up to us at
a craps table or something. When I learned this, I felt terrible for
missing out, but I knew I had made the right decision to cancel. Besides, Vegas doesn't seem like a great place to go with a suppressed
immune system. My brother spent the weekend there with them, so
it wasn't a total bust. But I was really sad to miss it, especially since

we don't get to see them very often anymore. I also backed out on the first annual trip to Six Flags with Heather's physics class. Clearly I was paying a price for these symptoms. In fact, it was while she was gone on that trip that my downward spiral really accelerated.

It all began with an afternoon of kite flying. Seems harmless enough, but one of my birthday presents was a dual-line stunt kite from Phil. This was not one of those little flappy kites with sticks and string; this was in a whole new league. It was basically a parachute about six feet wide, barely "tethered" to the planet with what I would consider to be a pair of small ropes, using me as a sort of elastic attachment medium. By elastic, I mean just barely anchored at best.

It was a moderately windy day by New Mexico spring standards, and I walked the block to campus to fly my new kite on the athletic field. It took some maneuvering to launch it from the end of the long lines, but after a couple tries I got it up. I was pretty cautious at first, not knowing how hard it would pull. Eventually, I got used to its feel and started to make some maneuvers, and after a while I became comfortable enough to get cocky. I let out a few extra feet of line and immediately paid the price. That was just enough length to allow it to rise above the tree line that protects the field from the higher winds, and it took off into the sky instantly. It literally lifted me off the ground. It dragged me by my wrists about forty feet across the grass with my toes barely scraping the ground as I hopelessly kicked for traction. At some point I managed to turn sideways enough to pull one cord harder than the other, sending the kite in a violent helical descent to the ground and landing me in a heap.

One arm had been hyper-extended by the sudden flight, which re-injured a shoulder dislocation from years past. I lay there on the grass and rolled over on my back to reposition my arm, laying it over my chest as I gazed into the clouds. I wiggled my hands out of the strings' wrist straps which had left scuff marks on the skin. I could feel the ache in my shoulder, throbbing with familiarity from the great pain of the original injury. What a bummer. I had worked diligently on that shoulder for six months in physical therapy, attempting to prevent this from happening again. All that work went down the tubes in a few short seconds.

I turned my head and surveyed the field to check if anyone had seen me. A guy walking his dog gave me a perplexed look from about fifty yards away. He must have gotten quite a show. I looked at him and waved my good arm to pretend like I was OK, and he wandered off. I lay there for a minute before sitting up. It had all happened so fast that I was in shock. *Holy crap, this kite is no toy,* I thought to myself. And I was right. I suppose it's no surprise that would be its one and only flight.

I climbed up off the ground and wadded up the cords, feeling too discombobulated to wind them properly (perhaps another reason why it's never flown again). I packed the whole kit back into its stuff sack, from which it has never re-emerged, and walked home. I had been feeling a bit run down before I went out, and now I was definitely exhausted. I was starting to get a thick, achy feeling in my throat, as though a head cold were coming. I probably shouldn't have gone out kite flying in the first place, but I wanted to enjoy some spring weather outside, sore throat or not.

That night I went to our neighbors' sixty-fourth birthday party. Of all our neighbors, past and present, they are our favorites. He's a retired professor, and she worked at the university as an administrator. They are really sharp people, but also very down to earth and fun to spend time with. We often got together for ice cream or a spontaneous dinner, just like friendly neighbors should do. Aside from enjoying close friendship with my parents, I've had very few good friends that much older than me, so it was really enjoyable to share with people who had such deep perspectives on life. Anyway, they had nearly the same birthday, so they celebrated it together. A few of their other friends joined us as well. We had dinner, talked about the old days, and we even sang the Beatles song apropos for the occasion.

By the time I got home, the achy swelling in my throat was really taking hold. I was starting to get feverish, and it seemed inevitable that I'd be getting sick. Heather returned late that night, but I was already in bed. The next day my sinuses began the most arduous three weeks they'd ever experienced. I'm prone to sinus infections due to my allergies and a deviated septum, so somewhere around half of my normal colds turned into bacterial infections. Actually that percentage is an improvement. Before I quit smoking,

I used to get an infection every time. Unfortunately, this one was really bad.

By day three, I was so miserable I couldn't sleep. My sinuses felt like a hot air balloon had been inflated inside every cavity. The pain and pressure were incredible. I was taking huge doses of acetaminophen, carefully avoiding NSAIDS [non-steroidal anti-inflammatory drugs (such as Ibuprofen and others)], as they're suspected of causing flares in IBD inflammation. I was bleary much of the time, being in great pain, and I wasn't getting any sleep. I had to keep a written record of the times and doses for my meds or I would forget when and what I had taken. I couldn't lay my head down, or the pain became unbearable, so I sat slouching back on the couch all night trying to sleep. A few times I may have dozed for a bit, but mostly I remember sitting there, in the dark, wrapped in a blanket, feeling absolutely miserable. I wanted to poke a hose into my cheeks to let out whatever was in there wreaking havoc.

I went to my primary doc who had no trouble diagnosing it as a sinus infection, and he gave me a prescription for Azithromycin, an antibiotic often referred to as a "Z-Pak." I didn't know it at the time, but that drug was a big no-no for folks like me. Worse yet, after ten days I hadn't improved, so I took an additional course of another type of antibiotic. Oops.

By then, desperate for help with my sinuses, I had also gone to see an Ear/Nose/Throat specialist. I got an MRI of my head, which clearly showed the nasty inflammation. But there wasn't much the specialist could do except recommend a daily regimen of steam tents, sinus irrigation, and Mucinex. This is when I discovered the magic Neil-Med sinus rinse system. It took another week before the pain receded and let me sleep at all, but by then I had developed a nasty cough.

After nearly a month of this misery, I slid into a funk from which I had a hard time imagining what it was like to feel well. And it wasn't only my sinuses. As I mentioned earlier, my colitis symptoms had been worsening over the previous weeks of high stress and reduced prednisone, and once I finished the second course of antibiotics my inflammation had roared back to the worst it had ever been and beyond.

I made a call to my GI doc, and they squeezed me in on short order. A sigmoidoscopy confirmed my fears that the situation was really bad. My colon was angrier than ever. Ulcers everywhere, horrible inflammation, and it went deeper than usual for me—all the way through the sigmoid colon, past my splenic flexure, and halfway across the transverse. So far in fact that the end was just beyond the reach of his 60cm scope-cam and he had to really cram it in to reach the end, not the easiest procedure we've been through together. I also had a strange abnormality near the anal opening, which he thought might be a fissure or a fistula. More on that later; for now let's call it the "anal artifact."

My gastroenterologist explained how broad-spectrum antibiotics have a habit of exacerbating IBD symptoms, something about a bacterial imbalance that lets some other bacteria called clostridium difficile cause problems. So, we tested for "c-diff," but it turned up negative. To this day, we're not totally sure what caused that flare-up, but it makes me extremely cautious about using antibiotics now (and getting in situations that require them). I was also coughing badly by then. He was worried I might be developing pneumonia and ordered some chest x-rays which turned up normal.

I felt extremely run down and very uncomfortable digestively. I was not eating well, and I moved quite slowly. I had lost more than fifteen pounds. He sent me home with orders to double my prednisone dosage and call him to report any developments. I spent most of my time in bed, too weak to go to work, save for the truly essential duties. I would teach my class and then hobble home immediately. Despite daily episodes of *Dr. Quinn* and back-to-back reruns of *Little House on the Prairie,* I was still quite miserable.

My situation did not improve. I left a message for my doctor a couple days later. He called back that afternoon, and we talked about options. We upped the prednisone again to my highest dosage ever. We knew my azathioprine dose was already at maximum because the metabolic tests showed that its toxic components in my system were approaching the warning range. I was also still taking large amounts of Asacol, which had never really worked since the first time. So I made a suggestion. My uncle had great things to say about the Mayo Clinic, where he went for help with Crohn's and liver problems. Perhaps I could benefit from another opinion or an alternate approach. Mayo, I pointed out, seems to be where people go (if they can) when they run out of other options. The doc agreed, somewhat to my surprise. He actually thought it was a good idea and seemed agreeable to cooperating with them on my treatment.

So I started making calls to Rochester, and the response I received was unlike anything I've ever experienced in the health care system. It was so amazing that it has its own chapter (coming up next). I got an appointment for just over a month away. But my health was not getting any better, and that was a long time to wait.

My doctor called a few days later to see how I was doing. In fact he called several times over that week. He was trying to decide if I needed to be hospitalized; if we couldn't get my acute symptoms under control, he would have no other choice. That was remarkable. I've never had a doctor call to look after me. Regardless of the practical side, I was deeply touched that he was watching out for me like that, and it really made me feel cared for. Such personal attention was uplifting to say the least. But it also made me very nervous. When a doctor calls you at home to check up on you, it means you're really sick. Prednisone, the one medicine that we could previously rely on, was no longer working, even at maximum human dosage, so things were looking pretty scary—especially since it wasn't clear to me what more they could do even if I were admitted to the hospital.

As a last ditch effort, he recommended that we try Rowasa. This is pretty much the same medicine as Asacol, only in liquid enema form. The idea is that it administers the drug directly to the affected area for people with left-sided colitis. Sounds lovely doesn't it?

OK. This might really work for some people, but I have to say that it was by far the hardest part of my treatment, bar none. An enema is not exactly a convenient procedure to perform on one's self. Take a quasi-squishable bottle of nasty stinging fluid with a prickly applicator tip; stick it where the sun doesn't shine and squeeze it till it's empty. This sounds easy enough, but then you gotta hold it all in. All night. How are you supposed to do that when you're asspissing every half hour? Plus, you'd think for two hundred bucks per six-pack they could come up with a bottle that's actually practical to use. Come on guys, how about a syringe-style applicator, or even a roll-up tube of some sort?

For better or worse, when I first started using Rowasa I had to sleep in another room by myself. I just couldn't be around another person under those circumstances. You probably know me by now; I'll share intimate details with all of you, but there's no way I was gonna get in bed with my wife and do that to myself. Actually I did adapt, but it was uncomfortable at best. Heather did her best to help me through it, but that was the epitome of my vulnerability. I don't think there's any way I could have felt better about it—it was just plain miserable.

Worst of all, it didn't seem to be working. I thought perhaps I perceived a minor improvement, but I wasn't sure. In any case, the fact that things weren't getting any worse was enough for my doctor to let me stay home. We did decide, however, that I couldn't wait much longer for a better solution, so I called and got my Mayo appointment moved up a week. Compared to almost all of my other experiences trying to get doctor appointments, the ease of dealing with the Mayo Clinic was a supportive reassurance. But that was only the beginning of what I would come to learn about Mayo. By then I only had two weeks to wait. We had originally planned the Mayo appointment to be after school was finished. But the new date meant we would now need to leave during Heather's final exam week. Her boss was sympathetic and helped her arrange to leave early.

The waiting period was a difficult time. My inflammation seemed to be stabilized—at a pretty bad level mind you, but it wasn't worsening. I still had a cough, which may have been attributable to my inactivity over the last month. One day my folks came to town. I'm not sure how premeditated it was, but they got me out of the house a bit. We went to the driving range, but I was too weak to enjoy it. We played some putting games for about an hour, and they took me home. This was the first time I'd been out of the house for anything not related to a doctor appointment or essential work obligation for several weeks. It felt good to do something normal.

Heather was exhausted too. I had been sleeping on a foam mattress in the living room so she could sleep at night without being burdened by my misery. She had to leave at five o'clock each morning for the eighty-mile commute to work. The stress of her first year teaching was challenging enough, and now I was in such bad shape. I don't have a vivid memory of how she dealt with it—she tends to confront things internally. She was helpful and supportive to me, but I was not in a good place and couldn't offer her much in return. Looking back, I can now appreciate the kind of heroics she showed.

It was during this time that the book you are now reading was conceived. I was sitting in the bathtub trying to soothe the "artifact" that had developed and feeling mostly miserable, but somehow at that moment I was still able to see humor in my condition. As I lay there soaking, I developed what would become the *Bionic Bunghole,* which I wrote later that night. I also dreamed up some of the other chapter titles and stories I would include. I wouldn't come to pick it up seriously, however, until two-and-a-half years later.

Finally the time arrived to make our Minnesota trek to the Mayo Clinic. I had enough frequent flyer miles to get a ticket, and my parents generously provided enough for Heather to come along. I'm so glad she did. It happens that my folks were also traveling up north that week for other obligations and were able to stop by and spend some time with us in Rochester.

One of my equipment vendors is located in Rochester as well, so through a contact there I found a great place for us to stay. It was a two-bedroom apartment above a storefront just a block from the clinic. It was on the skyway system, so there was no need to even go outside to get to my appointments, or to the mall next door, which had plenty of food available.

Under the assumption that I'd be undergoing some endoscopic procedures in the coming days, I was advised not to eat after 5 PM. This was made a tad difficult by the fact that there was a Greek restaurant directly beneath us, and the smell of gyros wafted up through our apartment (and continued to do so for our entire stay). Nevertheless, we hunkered down for the evening and anxiously awaited our upcoming big day.

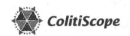

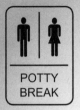

POTTY BREAK

During the school year, when Heather and I were living in separate cities, before the big flare-up started, I spent as many nights as I could in the city with her—we would drive together from her apartment to her school, and I'd meet up there with a carpool ride to my work.

During that stage it was common for me to make use of every bathroom I encountered. One of these mornings, while waiting for my ride, I went inside the teacher's lounge to use the restroom. While sitting in the stall, I noticed a peculiar piece of athletic tape on the wall with writing on it. I leaned over to read it. To my great surprise, it was a bomb threat! I had visions of that *Lethal Weapon* movie with a bomb beneath the toilet and instinctively peered under my throne, looking for anything suspicious. I found nothing. It occurred to me that someone ought to know about this, so I quickly finished my task and headed for the office. I explained who I was and what I had found. They thanked me and asked for my cell number in case anyone would need to follow up.

I heard nothing more about it until Heather got home from work. Maggie, a friend far away in Minnesota, whose job is to scan local stories on the newswire for publication, had come across a story about this bomb threat at the school where Heather works. Of course she called Heather right away. Maggie was intrigued to learn that I was the one who had found the note. Thankfully, in the end it turned out to be an empty threat, and nothing became of it aside from our little small-world connection. But it was all over the local news that night. If only all those people who heard about the incident knew that it was discovered because I had an emergency poop! Yep, an unlikely and unrecognized hero once again.

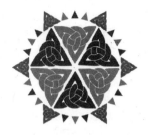

Please Pass the Mayo

And Whip Me Up a Miracle

Standing in the lobby of the Mayo Clinic makes a person feel regal. It's a huge, bright, open area nearly as large as the main building itself, covered in butterscotch marble with twenty-foot ceilings. The entire east wall has floor-to-ceiling windows and glass doors, with wide terraced stairs leading down from the museum-like entrance. It's less hospital and more Hyatt hotel than any clinic I've ever been to. Heavy brass stanchions with crimson velvet ropes loosely suggest a path for the line to form, which stretches from the reception area out into the open lobby, drenched in spring sunrise.

There's a microcosm of humanity weaving through this hall, representing a diverse macro-culture. Each person in line clearly has a story, a long one. Each clings to an armful of medical records, x-ray envelopes, catalogues of lab tests, physician dictations, and evidence of whatever else they have tried in desperation before they landed here, by whatever means. Each of these people represents a human drama stretched to its thinnest, pushed to the edge, brought to its knees. A gaze around this room would humble even the sickest person.

Every ethnicity I can imagine is represented here, every age and social status, and a multitude of languages. The translation department here must rival the U.N. offices in New York. Some patients have partners, others stand alone. I can only imagine their thoughts. I have true love by my side, the power of which holds me up, and I feel for those without. I feel also for those who suffer and don't find themselves here. Most people here dress as though they have the resources to make their visit possible. Suddenly I am aware of how fortunate I am to be here, to have this beacon of hope.

I have made this journey in a time of desperation—my symptoms uncontrollable, my future threatened. We must all be at such a juncture to have ended up here. And so the weight of collective burden borne by this group gathered in the lobby shows its heaviness, especially when I consider that this and every Monday morning there's a new line just like this one, a never-ending supply of raw humanity streaming through this place, a gateway to last hope.

Everything here is handled with class. A polite attendant checks with everyone in line, ensuring that we're all in the right place. The line moves smoothly; registration is efficient; and we are on our way upstairs sooner than I thought possible. Columns of elevators whisk people to all parts of the complex. Specialists in every imaginable ailment are tucked somewhere inside this buzzing machine. We board the elevator with a collection as diverse as we'd seen in line. Some young and bald, others old and frail, all speechless and pensive. Regardless of how sick I may be, I see what some others here are struggling with and easily decide I can be happy with my disease. Compared to what I could have, I'll take what I've got.

As clever as this place may be, it strikes me as a bit odd to have the gastrointestinal department on nearly the top floor. It's a long ride to be trapped without a bathroom. Even stranger, we exit on the GI floor and see a sign for a memorial conference room dedicated to Dr. Hugh Butt. No joke.

Our wait is short, and we are taken to an exam room promptly at appointment time. The room looks to be lifted right out of a Frank Lloyd Wright project. Mid-century linear design with a touch of deco, it has a wooden floor with a tight parquet pattern of end-grain maple. The walls are covered with vertical wooden slats of varied thicknesses, and a built-in desk and bookshelf adorn the windowed wall at the far end. A comfy settee lines one side of the room where we are invited to relax while we wait. I sit and gaze at the exam table, which is made of solid wood with dovetailed corners in a rich walnut finish, cleverly infused with cabinets and drawers. It is truly a work of art.

This place was built of a time and attitude not common in modern architecture. Care and expense were undertaken to make each and every room an artful reflection of the quality that lies within and throughout. It's refreshing for me as an artist and engineer to witness such attention to something I thought we'd lost with the rise of bottom-line capitalism—the integration and celebration of both function and form. One can only assume that such an aura of beauty and craftsmanship would naturally invoke an environment for quality work and care. By osmosis they would encourage each other. It feels like a magical synergy, and it comforts me.

The central strategy of a Mayo visit is to put together a team of specialists who coordinate to get all the tests and procedures they need to make a diagnosis. For most patients this process takes three or four days; then you meet again with your advisory team, discuss the prognosis, and formulate a treatment plan. Sometimes that plan requires further work at the clinic; often it is a program that accompanies you home to be implemented with your own doctor.

My first appointment was mostly a condition history done by a physician's assistant. She asked a lot of questions, patiently listened to my story, and gathered relevant items from the records I'd brought along. Toward the end of the session, the doctor came to discuss it all with us. We made a list of tests to procure and talked about the concerns we had. He left and we finished up with the P.A. She said we'd meet again on Wednesday for a debriefing.

"This Wednesday, as in two days from now?" I asked in disbelief.

"Yes, at three in the afternoon, two days from now." She replied, acknowledging my surprise, "We have a schedule for you." She led us out of the room to the administrative desk where we were assigned our own personal scheduling specialist. The P.A. said goodbye and left us in the hands of a miracle worker.

"Here's your schedule Mr. Tubesing, everything you need is in here, and my phone number is on the front. If you have any questions about the schedule or the preparations, or if you have any

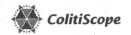

problems at all, call me at this number. If I'm not in, someone else will be able to help you, twenty-four hours a day."

"Wow," I said, taking the packet from her. It was like an airplane ticket folder; inside there was a stack of appointment cards, all in chronological order, with the first one sticking through a slot in the front of the folder. My next appointment, for blood tests, was coming up in fifteen minutes. The next few cards for the first day were for several MRIs and an administrative appointment for billing and orientation. The next two days included a colonoscopy, barium x-rays, a Mantoux test (to check for TB in case we decide to try a new medicine called Remicade), and a few other examinations. Amazing. It would have taken me a month to arrange just one of those appointments back home, and accomplishing it all would have taken the whole summer.

The next two days were a flurry of appointments and logistics. First I had blood tests, taken by a very cheery young woman. Then followed a series of MRI imaging, a colonoscopy, and some x-rays taken with a belly full of barium (a half gallon of liquid chalk they made me drink). Not one of these procedures was performed by a technician; they were all done by gastroenterologists and radiologists. I have never had an M.D. perform some of those procedures. It was amazing. The person who was responsible for reading the results was the person performing the tests. They had direct interaction with the imaging process.

During my MRI, the doc came in and asked about my anal artifact (the thing we thought might be a fissure or fistula) because he couldn't see it on the screen. He moved me around a bit and tried other approaches until he found it. The x-ray procedure was done by a radiology M.D. who was looking at real-time pictures for signs of Crohn's inflammation or damage in my small intestine. I was strapped to a motorized articulating table so he could tilt me to any angle he needed. He kept poking my belly with a long prod, trying to move the contrast fluid through me. The colonoscopy was performed by a pair of M.D.'s, one a seasoned expert, the other a surgical resident. They were not accustomed to conducting this procedure with a conscious patient, so I think it was a little strange for them. I could hear the mentor guiding his resident through some of the tricky parts, like coercing the scope into the ileum at the end of the colon, and collecting the biopsy samples.

Everyone we came into contact with was extremely professional, dressed well, and emanated an overwhelming sense that they enjoyed what they do and took it seriously—all the nurses, the blood collectors, even the receptionists. It was a five-star experience for sure. Plus the environment was second to none. While waiting for the blood tests I gazed around the room and noticed on the wall what looked like a huge Joan Miró print. I got up for a closer look and realized that there were actually three, a triptych of prints, each about six feet tall and two feet wide. I thought they were awfully big for reprints, but as I approached I noticed visible brush strokes and an autograph in pencil. These were not prints; they were Joan Miró originals. Holy moly! This place is like a museum. I'd heard that hospitals have their own curators, but this was not normal hospital artwork; this stuff could be on the walls of MOMA. Later I found a multi-panel Andy Warhol original in the cafeteria hallway and another piece by my favorite sculptor, Harry Bertoia, in an elevator lobby. What an amazing place to spend a few days.

It's nice that they gave me such a clear schedule because it mitigated some interesting timing challenges. I had to fast forty-eight hours for Tuesday's colonoscopy, but Wednesday's x-rays only for twelve, so if I finished the colonoscopy by six that evening, I could eat one meal before fasting again. Fasting also included staying off my meds during that time, so I had a welcome break from the pharmaceutical buffet—except the prednisone, which they let me ingest because you can't stop taking it suddenly. Oh joy.

All in all we completed an incredible amount of medical data gathering in those two-and-a-half days. Heather sat in waiting rooms a lot and read books. Surprisingly, even with all those appointments in different places, I hardly had to wait at all. I had wanted to talk with a dietitian during my time there, which is normal for GI patients, but for whatever reason, that was the one appointment they couldn't squeeze in for me.

We met Wednesday afternoon for the debriefing. The P.A. was there again, along with the GI doc we'd seen on Monday, and a colorectal surgeon who came to offer consultation on surgical options. As this is a teaching hospital, there were also a few observers, GI and surgical residents I suspect. Discussions centered on the debate over my diagnosis. Do I have Crohn's disease or ulcerative colitis? There wasn't a clear consensus because my anal artifact presented a puzzle. After all the evaluation I'd gone through those three days, nobody would even have suspected Crohn's because the indicators didn't show up anywhere but my lower colon...except for that odd fissure/fistula mystery, and even it was way down in my rectum.

A fistula appears when your body, for whatever bizarre reason, by inflammation carves itself a passageway from the digestive tract (usually the small or large intestine) to a new place. Sometimes they lead to other parts of the GI system; sometimes they open up into the abdominal cavity; and sometimes they tunnel all the way to the skin surface, as in my case. Weird! Fistulas are definitely more of a Crohn's symptom than colitis, but a few rare people do get them without having IBD at all. Was it possible that by some fluke I had gotten it for an unrelated reason? It's hard to know.

The surgeon was the most curious about it and seemed more convinced than the others it was an indicator of Crohn's disease. There was also some speculation that it might be a simple fissure (sort of like a split lip on the anus). I showed him the pictures from my first colonoscopy a few years earlier and he saw something we hadn't noticed up to that point. The same artifact they were concerned about showed up in the picture from years back. We didn't even have to look closely to see it. How could we have missed that before? How could the original surgeon who did that procedure not have noticed it, especially having photographed it? We were all bewildered.

"Drop your pants," the surgeon suddenly suggested, "Let's have a look at it." So he and the other two docs and the interns all peered around my backside to see the circus show. I've never done that in front of a group before, but at this point I had pretty much lost all need for modesty in these situations. I heard the familiar snap of exam gloves and felt some very odd sensations.

"That's definitely a fistula," the surgeon insisted, crossing the room to throw away his gloves, "Let's do surgery tomorrow."

"Tomorrow?" I asked in disbelief.

"Yep, come to the outpatient surgery center at seven tomorrow morning, we'll do surgery at eight."

I was dumbfounded. Is it even possible to do a surgery on fifteen hours notice? Sure, in an emergency, but I've never heard of arranging an elective surgery on that kind of time line. Can he schedule it like that without an array of phone calls? This place is truly exceptional.

He explained about the surgery, what they would do, and how it should help the fistula heal. They would install a "seton," which is sort of a rubber string that they thread through the fistula tunnel, into the rectum, and back out through the anus. It would then get looped around to the entry point and tied off on the outside. This approach is supposed to help the fistula drain and heal from the inside so it stays closed permanently rather than continually healing on the surface with festering infection trapped inside.

So the next morning I had surgery. It was that simple, save for yet another fast. Though of course, I was quite nervous. As you may recall, I don't even like the sedation for a colonoscopy, and this was general anesthesia and surgery, so the anxiety was plentiful. But I was able to keep calm somehow. My folks came down from Wisconsin to keep us company, and it was very nice to have them nearby. Before going in, I gave Heather a long kiss and told her that in case of the unthinkable, my ashes should be packed into blue fireworks and shot off over the harbor in our hometown. It made her cry.

I got wheeled through a series of holding areas and prep rooms until finally I came to the operating room. The anesthesiologist was quite nice and calming. We chatted a little about the procedure and what I'd experience. After one last confirmation of my name, birth date, and the purpose for surgery, they started my shut-down process. I was nervous, but they seemed very competent.

As one last effort to ease my nerves, I called out to everyone in the room, "Hey everybody, do a good job today."

They chuckled, and I fell asleep. Somehow it seemed that reminding them it's a real and vulnerable person they're working on today seemed like a good idea, not that they really needed the reminder, but I hoped it would make me seem like a person rather than a project. It made me feel better anyway.

I awoke in the recovery room seemingly a moment later. I was groggy but not in pain. After an hour or so of re-orienting myself

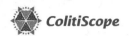

and attention from a nurse, I drank some fluids and got dressed. The nurse and I met with Heather, and she gave us the discharge instructions—basically they told me to stay put for twenty-four hours, ease back into food, and call with any problems. I rested the remainder of the day and went to bed early.

When I got up the next morning, I had the strangest kind of pain and discomfort. It felt like every muscle in my body was aching badly from exercise. I was totally fatigued, as if I'd played a football game yesterday (and lost badly, to a much bigger team). And I mean every muscle was sore and weak. I finally got a chance to buy those Gyros I'd been smelling for several days and couldn't even pinch a dollar bill with my thumb and index finger, it fell to the ground. Not sure if this was normal, we called the surgeon's office. He called back and explained, "If you'd seen the positions we had you in yesterday you wouldn't be so surprised." He described the awkward-sounding postures I underwent during surgery, and some of my discomfort seemed more sensible. He also explained that the muscle weakness could be a residual effect of the anesthesia and that I shouldn't be concerned if it didn't last more than a day.

I was starting to get a little stir crazy in our empty apartment. It hadn't been twenty-four hours yet since the surgery, but we were supposed to go home the next day, and I hadn't been to Fleet Farm yet—which I never miss a chance to visit because there's nothing like it where we live now. Billed as "The Man's Mall," it's sort of a home improvement center, tractor/farm supply, five-and-dime, and sportsmen's warehouse, all under one roof. So that's the one rule I broke while I was there, braving a trip out during the post-surgical rest period for some man-style shopping. No surprise that I didn't feel well once I got there and had to return (empty-handed) for a nap. I got what I deserved for trying to over-rule the surgeon's discharge orders.

I must say the seton they installed created a very odd situation, basically resulting in a pierced perineum for a couple months until the wound healed and the seton fell out, sort of like stitches or a splinter that the body pushes out as it heals. My anal artifact had been converted into a bunghole bowtie, and it felt quite strange. Being an open wound, things were a bit messy down there for a while. I found a good solution for that problem but there was definitely a learning curve—if I were to write a chapter on that topic alone, it would be titled "Manly Pads: A Gentlemen's Guide to Mastering the Maxi."

A final consult with the docs concluded that I should seriously consider Remicade once I got home. The GI doc on my team was the lead researcher on the Humira trials, so they talked about that as a future possibility. It had already been approved for Rheumatoid Arthritis, but the IBD applications were still in study. Remicade and Humira are a newer class of medications for immune system disorders; more on that later. It was reassuring to get the scoop, not from someone who was merely familiar with the latest news, but from someone who was making the headlines—all contributing to my lasting impression of what an amazing place the Mayo Clinic is.

There still wasn't a lot of certainty about my diagnosis, though the surgeon remained more sure than the others. We settled on "indeterminate colitis," and that's how it's been ever since. Eventually the fistula healed (and never returned), but even more important, my inflammation symptoms improved remarkably quickly. In fact I was mystified by how fast I sprung back in the following days— especially since I hadn't received any treatments or medications while I was there, save for the surgery, which did not explain the dramatic reduction of inflammation inside my colon. In hindsight, we are fairly certain that the trigger for my sudden progress was that I hadn't been taking my normal medications during those days at Mayo. For the first time since I'd gone back on Asacol two years earlier, I got a break from it. My home doctor and I now theorize that I may be one of those few whose symptoms are worsened by that drug. That explained a lot, so I stayed off it.

Additionally, since my symptoms were improving so dramatically, we decided not to change anything else. We didn't want to risk losing that progress so we left my medication plan as it had been, but without the Asacol, keeping just prednisone and azathioprine. My colon has been quite stable ever since. I haven't had a major flare since then, though I can only get the prednisone down to a certain level before my symptoms sneak back. So maybe it's time to consider other options, and now we're talking about Remicade once again, but that's another story.

Looking back on my experience at the Mayo Clinic, I am both amazed and humbled. It was incredibly helpful, and I feel very fortunate to have been able to go there. It was an extraordinary environment in which to receive medical attention; the care was truly exceptional; and it was highly effective.

Adding to my overall amazement was the bill that came a week later. Rather than the typical situation where everybody and their brother sends a separate indecipherable invoice, everything I did at Mayo and associated facilities came together on one single bill! All very easy to understand, and at an incredibly reasonable price. I was left in awe.

I wouldn't promise you a miracle, but if your circumstances ever get as confusing and frightening as mine did, and if you can somehow manage to do it, go there. I have nothing to gain from suggesting this to you, so rest assured that I say it with purest intent.

Of course that advice is based on my particular experience in a place that worked great for me. Really, the most important challenge for each of us is that we find a resource where we feel we're really listened to, where we get the answers we need, and where we are truly cared for. You may find that supportive resource to be the doctor you currently see, and if so then consider yourself blessed. Otherwise, keep looking until you get what you need. We all deserve quality health services, and we're paying customers, so we don't have to settle for inadequate care.

Part II

Scope & Cope

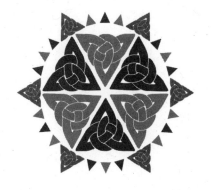

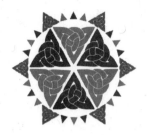

Bathrooms 101

There's so much to talk about on the bathroom topic, especially for those with IBD. We experience restrooms with such intensity that we have become absolute authorities on the topic. Let these thoughts be fun and practical advice for those with IBD, something educational for those who know and love us, and a mandate for those who create and control these places in which we spend so much of our time.

Here are the most likely places to find a...

Clean bathroom:

Downtown: Upscale hotel lobby. If anyone asks, just tell them you're staying there. Sometimes the facilities are far away from the entrance through a grand hall, so a hotel may not be the best choice if you're on a Nature 911 call, but if you can make it through the lobby, then you'll be going in style. Marble décor, cloth towels, sometimes even free aftershave— and if you're really lucky, the soothing *Girl from Ipanema* will gently accompany your stay.

On the road: Chain restaurant

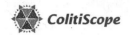

In general: Home! Aside from these suggestions on finding actual restrooms, IBD folks know that just about anything qualifies to be a toilet now and again. Trash cans, buckets, bushes, even a grocery bag—all can do the job if need be.

Nasty bathroom:

Downtown: A bar. Avoid this at all costs, Chinese restaurants and urban gas stations too.

On the road: Truck stop. Yes they'll have plenty of stalls, but they'll definitely be nasty. Though on the plus side, truck stops often have showers you can rent, so that's the place to go if you're suffering from premature evacuation.

In general: Grocery stores. I swear their bathrooms are intentionally disgusting and inaccessible so nobody will use them.

Bathroom with an available stall:

Airport: Head for one close to an unoccupied departure gate.

Department store: Technically this doesn't count because you're not likely to find the bathroom at all, but if you do find yourself looking, the children's clothing department is a good place to start, and remember there are still some old-school stores that have fewer men's than women's rooms, and they're sometimes located in completely different parts of the store.

High school: Maybe times have changed, and perhaps it's a guy thing, but where I went to school, NOBODY used the toilet stalls, and nowadays they rarely have doors for fear of condoning illicit activity. So if you find yourself stuck in a high school, try the locker room, it's usually unoccupied during the day and probably the most socially acceptable place in school to take a dump. If this is a real issue for you, try lobbying for approval to use the teacher's bathroom or another more private facility.

Truck stop: Yep, they have lots of stalls, but it won't be a pretty sight.

Bathroom without an available stall:

Starbucks: Sometimes they only have one bathroom, but if not, the men's and women's will both be one-holers. If your gender is occupied it's OK to use the other; you have a digestive handicap which affords you this option. Don't be shy.

Bathrooms with the most pee on the seats:

Bars: Beer, duh.

Rock concerts: In this case it's more likely puke.

Sporting events: Beer, duh, again.

Bathrooms you'll never reach in time:

Shopping malls: Hands down, bar none. If you have to take a crap at the mall you might as well walk to the car instead of the bathroom because you're going home for a shower either way.

Bathrooms with footprints on the seats:

Places where they don't sit on the toilet: Any Middle Eastern, African, or Asian country or western locations frequented by these cultures. Turkish toilets are typical in these places, so when you do find a western toilet, often it will have footprints on it from those who use it Turkish style.

A bathroom that you can't fit in:

An RV: For whatever reason, the designers of these expensive homes-on-wheels think the last place they should spend floor space on is the bathroom. Even the fancy ones have crappers that make a phone booth look palatial. Why is this? Isn't the motor home market aimed primarily at retirees? Aren't they the population most affected by health issues? So why on earth should it be so hard to find a camper with a bathroom that's big enough to actually close the door when you're sitting on the toilet? Worse yet

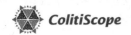

are the designs that integrate the toilet and shower so you have to straddle the bowl while showering, making everything wet. Though I guess there's a bright side for people like us who get the runs all the time, we don't have to exit the shower to relieve ourselves! One day some designer will wake up and realize that there are people who might actually want a luxurious bathroom in their camper, and we'll finally get a reasonable space to do our business.

Too much politics wrapped up in the bathroom:

Santa Fe, New Mexico. First of all, low-flow (AKA no-flushey-the-stuffy) toilets are required everywhere in the state; it is illegal for a plumber to install a toilet that is actually capable of flushing properly. But here's the kicker: To acquire building permits involving bathrooms, for every toilet installed in the project, the builder must purchase and install a minimum of eight additional toilets elsewhere to replace older models. I shit you not; you get one for the price of nine. So for every nine toilets that would have worked fine, now there are nine that don't. It is noteworthy to mention that as this concept was being implemented, eight percent of the Santa Fe municipal water supply was being consumed by a single golf course. Forgive me for appearing presumptuous here, but if you're in a water crisis and a seven-year drought, maybe you should be golfing on brown grass instead of making everybody flush three times. Note how every toilet in the southwest has a plunger next to it and how in more sensible states this is not the case. Figure it out guys.

❊ ❊ ❊

Seriously, finding a restroom while out in public is typically not an easy task, and when the need arises, this search immediately becomes serious business for us. Most businesses have bathrooms because, at the very least, their employees need access, but many are hesitant to let the public use them. I can understand that. After all they have to clean it, and the less use it gets the less cleaning it needs.

Generally in these cases I have found most people to be sympathetic if I am polite and appear to be genuinely in need. The Crohn's and Colitis Foundation provides a membership card when you join, and the back side of the card is meant as a bathroom pass (I call it the "Ass Pass"). It explains concisely that the bearer of the card has a medical condition that requires speedy bathroom access. I have found it useful on occasion. I have also succeeded by saying things like, "I understand your hesitation, but could I please appeal to your sense of mercy here; I am truly in need." I have also been prepared to offer a free bathroom cleaning when I'm done, which I figure might be enough motivation to offer an exception to their policy, but it hasn't been necessary yet. Sometimes a simple reassurance that you're a regular, or that you'll make a purchase, will do the trick— in which case it's a good idea to follow through.

When I get a snide, stubborn, or uncooperative response, I sometimes fantasize about what I could say. *Gotta be a customer eh? Well why would I ever want to become your customer if you won't let me use the bathroom?* or *Let's hope you never have the need in my place of business,* or *Take your pick, either let me use it or I'll lose it right here on your Ralph Lauren carpet.* Of course those approaches would never work and don't seem to generate the sort of karma we need, so best to keep them to one's self.

In any case, we need to respect a favor when it is offered. Always leave such a restroom cleaner than you found it. Try not to clog the toilet and fix it if you do. Use their air freshener if they have some. In general, help them to not regret what they have done for you and they'll be more inclined to extend this courtesy to the next person.

There are plenty of other situations where solutions are less apparent. These sometimes require a bit of creativity, and the more experience you get, the more honed your radar will become. My wife and I walk around the neighborhood fairly often. I have never needed to, but at times I've considered knocking on a stranger's door. So far I have always found another option. For instance, there's a house being remodeled on the block over from us. They have a porta-potty in the yard for the construction workers to use, and I have made use of it myself. I plan my walks so it can serve as a midway backup facility. I've done the same at other construction sites.

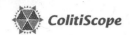

Such an option is not always available of course, and at times a make-shift biffy must be improvised. We IBD sufferers become accustomed to observing so much more than your average person. Screen shots from the Terminator's viewpoint pop to mind—robotic computer vision, constantly scanning the landscape, analyzing data, identifying, highlighting, and cataloging adaptable solutions at every step.

Some people are tempted to ask me, how on earth do I survive an eighty-mile commute to work? Well, there are several answers to that question. Mostly, it's made possible by keeping my symptoms under control. If I had a major flare-up, this would be much more difficult, but luckily, since I started driving this long haul on a daily basis I have been relatively healthy. Knock on wood. I have found the best way to manage my commute on a daily basis is to eat strategically. I always allow at least 20 minutes after eating before I get in the car; otherwise I wait to eat breakfast until I get to work. My other strategy is that, after making the drive about six hundred times, I know the mile marker of every bathroom enroute. I always know exactly how far it is to the nearest gas station, motel lobby, rest area, and other pit stop possibilities. But it's a long drive across an empty desert, so the stops are few and far between. For this reason, I also know where to find all the dry creek beds and culverts big enough to hide in along the way—though these are B.Y.O.BW. facilities, which require a little more preparation. So I always have a roll of TP somewhere in the car and, when symptoms warrant, a packet of tissues in my pocket.

But proximity is not the only issue. Others can often be confused or even offended by my sudden needs, especially if they're not familiar with my routine. Sometimes I have to end phone calls prematurely or simply disappear in the middle of a conversation. I assume that when people who know me are involved they'll help smooth things over, but to some people I must end up looking quite rude—in which case I either try to offer a hasty explanation as I run down the hall or fill them in when I return.

How do I handle this issue as a teacher, standing in front of a class for fixed periods, you ask? Of course, carefully timing my meals and snacks is the first step, as usual. Second, there's typically a bathroom close enough if I can get moving in time. So, to facilitate an easy departure, on all my lecture notes the side bar is scattered with contextual questions or tasks I can quickly pose to my students to work on while I make a run for it. Occasionally I've had to bolt with minimal warning. Then I apologize when I return and get on with the material. Hard as this may be to imagine, it doesn't cause much disruption; students are generally pretty tolerant.

I'm glad, however, that I don't share my wife's situation; in the building where she does most of her teaching, the restrooms are in a separate section accessible only by going outside, which means a long walk to get there. Plus, after school hours the entry hallway is locked, and she doesn't have a key. I simply couldn't work there, and I'm confused about how this could possibly be legal. How can an isolated cluster of nine classrooms not have a bathroom? Her other classroom is a little better—it has an adjacent bathroom shared with the shop class next door, but it's rarely equipped with supplies and, in typical high school fashion, the stall has no door and the exterior door does not lock. Unfortunately, this is not unusual nowadays. Many districts have revoked bathroom privacy in an effort to curb bathroom mischief. I really feel for high school kids with IBD; their lives are definitely not easy.

Actually getting to the bathroom is one challenge, but there are a host of other possible roadblocks as well: crowded bathrooms, dirty/abused/broken facilities, insufficient supplies, un-private restroom designs, and I'm sure you can think of many more.

In a public situation where you're faced with waiting in line for a stall, I highly recommend simply explaining to those waiting that you have an urgent situation. Call it a digestive handicap. Flash your Ass Pass. You might be surprised how understanding people can be. *Everybody* has experienced a memorable bathroom emergency, so you have that to your advantage.

As for toilet seats with pee on them, I seriously want to piss on the people who do that. I mean, come on, is it really *that* much trouble to lift the lid? Don't want to touch it? Fine, use your brain: lift it with the sole of your shoe. I have no sympathy for whatever need that person perceived there to be for pissing on the seat. There's no valid excuse. Even if it was an accident, they should have the courtesy to clean up after themselves.

On a slightly more challenging note, there really are some places nobody would want to go to the bathroom. Some restrooms are so disgusting that I can hardly bring myself to enter, let alone touch anything. Indeed, there are times when I risk soiling myself and walk out of these places without using them. It makes me angry. Sometimes I want to defile these places further, so the person who left the mess would have to sleep in the bed they made. But they're never the ones who are left to deal with it. Most likely it will be some underpaid teenager at the bottom of the seniority ladder who gets the clean-up job. Or somebody else; it doesn't matter; *nobody* wants to deal with a mess like that, whether it's their job or not. And so I imagine the next person coming after me to be someone with needs like mine, and I end up trying to leave every restroom I use cleaner than I found it.

There are times, however, when you have no alternative but to cause further damage. Twice I've had to leave a load on top of a hopelessly clogged toilet because I had no other choice. One of those times was in a restaurant with only a single uni-sex bathroom, and there were several people waiting in line to use it after me. I had waited longer than I thought I was capable of to get in there; then, upon finding it inoperable, I felt more stuck than ever before. The plunger didn't work, the bowl was nearly overflowing, but it came down to using it or my pants, and I was far enough from home to exclude the pants possibility. I paced around inside, crowning, trying to imagine an alternative, and failed. So I had to do it, and I added to the mess. I felt awful. I tried to explain to the next person in line, but it was hard to do without looking them in the eye. It was a true "Ben Stiller" moment; only it wasn't just something to cringe about at the movies, this was really happening. The remaining ten minutes in the restaurant waiting for the check were excruciating. It was a small open eating area with no place to hide. I felt bad for those in line as well, but I couldn't take the full blame. It's just plain irresponsible to have only a single toilet to serve an entire restaurant. Frankly I don't understand how that can meet building codes. Maybe it doesn't; I certainly hope not.

For the sake of preparation, it's important to think of all the potential solutions before you're in urgent need. Make sure you're well-equipped to deal with any urgency or accident. Often we're not thinking clearly in those situations so some forethought will be worth the effort. Know where to look for a real bathroom, and how to create one of your own. In isolated places it's easier to find privacy in the bush, so supplies will be essential. For those cases be sure you have some tissues along at all times (and some wet wipes or hand sanitizer too).

Even when you're well, you want to be prepared all the time—you never know when you (or a companion) might need supplies. Those in deciduous geographies have the option of gathering leaves in an emergency, but since I live in the desert, one word can guarantee that I'll never be caught without other options: *Cactus*. Even if you live in a foliage-filled area, there are good reasons to carry your own supplies. If you doubt me, read the ice fishing story in this book *(Ice Hole)*. Right now, go read it; you can come back to this section later.

The obvious solution is to carry an emergency kit. I have several types that I use for different purposes. My brother coined the term *Shit Kit* but *Fanny Pack* will do for a family-friendly nickname.

There's a bare-bones kit that I carry in my pocket when symptoms are dicey. It has a travel pack of Kleenex, a plastic bag, and a few individually packaged wet wipes. This is enough to get me through most tricky situations, and ensures I'll never be under-supplied in a bathroom or make-shift facility.

There's a slightly better equipped version in my brief case which is rarely more than a hundred feet away. This one has the same stuff as the mini-kit, in larger quantities, in addition to a compressed magic towel and a change of underwear. The magic towel is a pretty clever item. It is a small cloth towel compressed into a little pill shape, about twice as thick as a Life Saver (and that's exactly what they can be). Just add water and presto, instant washcloth. I put all this stuff into a little zipper bag so it's easy to grab and go. I keep one in my golf bag too.

There's also a complete emergency kit in my office. A trusted friend knows the location of it. This one has everything mentioned previously, but adds a pair of pants as well. Obviously this complete kit is for the most extreme cases. Thankfully I've never had to use it, but it eases my mind knowing it's there, especially eighty miles

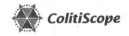
from home. I should really keep one of these in the trunk of my car as well, but I haven't gotten around to that yet.

I have assembled these kits in what they call "Pack-it Cubes." Adventure outfitters like REI typically carry them. They're fabric zipper bags meant for sub-dividing your clothes for easy packing. They have handles and come in several sizes. One of mine is just the right size for a pair of pants and a bunch of supplies. I also have another about half that size, which I use for a summer kit with a pair of shorts. It's a nice way to make a non-descript package that someone could fetch for you without even knowing what's inside. Plus, this is a great way for me to utilize some of the underwear I bought and didn't like enough to put in regular rotation.

If you're a friend, family member, or someone who spends a lot of time with an IBD patient, it would be a very thoughtful gesture for you to consider adding some or all of these supplies to your own traveling accessories. At some point you may very well save the day. And who knows, you might even end up using it yourself. *Be Prepared.*

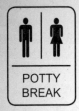

POTTY BREAK

The summer before I was originally diagnosed with colitis, we undertook a wiring project at home. We added communications wiring to the entire house for telephones, computer network, cable TV and even surround speakers. It was cheap and easy for me, having been in the communications contracting business, so we put several jacks in each room to be sure there would be plenty.

Perhaps still exhibiting our family tendency for the over-kill approach to projects, I had planned to put a phone jack in the master bathroom. I thought it might be handy on occasion. My wife and brother, who were helping on the project, thought I was nuts. They gave me so much grief about it, mostly in jest, that I finally scrapped the idea to save time and materials.

As much as I'd love to be gracious in retrospect, instead I have only one thing to say to them: *I told you so!*

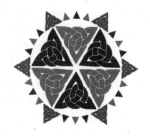

But You Don't Look Sick

Here's a conversation I'm sure we've all participated in, at one level or another:

"I heard/wondered/noticed that you have some health problems..."

"Yeah, I have Inflammatory Bowel Disease."

"Oh, Irritable Bowel Syndrome? My brother-in-law gets that sometimes; he can't eat Ethiopian food."

We politely explain that while IBS is definitely a challenging condition, IBD is different. It is not an illness that we can escape by avoiding ethnic foods or staying away from dairy products. Of course, we empathize and share many challenges with sufferers of all bowel ailments, but at the same time, we prefer to be understood for our specific situation.

"Inflammatory bowel disease is an immune disorder in which your body attacks its digestive organs like a transplant patient's body sometimes rejects the replacement organ as if it were a foreign invasion. Diet certainly affects my symptoms, but it doesn't have a causal relationship with the illness."

"Oh, oh my, is that serious?"

"Yes, it's a chronic disease."

"But you don't look sick."

This is a classic illustration of a significant, yet hidden, IBD challenge—that we truly do have a handicap, but it doesn't look like it from the outside. In some sense that's good. In order to feel OK about our situation, we do an excellent job of hiding it, at least in appearance. However, when interacting with the outside world, we don't have crutches, limps, prosthetics, or other symptoms and accessories that would alert others to our limitations (or if we do, we conceal them rigorously). We also commonly don't have observable physical characteristics that people associate with the chronically ill; we don't outwardly look like we're suffering. But that doesn't mean we couldn't benefit from some understanding accommodations when needed.

Sometimes at the store I need to park close to the entrance so I can make it to the bathroom quickly. But imagine what would happen if I used a handicap space. Regardless of whether I had a permit or not, people would see me jump out of my car and run inside, which is hardly the sort of behavior a disabled person engages in. Resentment would be natural, I admit it; I've had those thoughts too. A kid who looks like he borrowed grandma's car to run to the store appears to be taking advantage of her handicap parking permit. Sure, I've cursed all those empty spaces right up front that seem excessive in size and quantity. But I gotta say that many times I have wished for a blue placard on my rear-view mirror so I could have a head start running for the can. On top of that, there's a host of places that carefully control the use of their restrooms. Can you imagine if they kept their handicap parking spaces or wheelchair ramp under lock and key? They'd be shut down.

This came to issue for me a couple years ago when my wife and I chaperoned her science club's trip to an amusement park. It was "Physics Day," and the park was closed to all but physics students so they could explore science in action. It was truly a microcosm— the nerdiest bunch of kids I'd ever seen, all running around with notebooks, calculators, and accelerometers, which on any other day would make them stick out like super-geeks. However, because it was only them on that day, they were all super-cool instead.

Anyway, I generally don't enjoy those kinds of places because bathrooms are usually crammed in corners that you can never find, and the chances of getting there in time are pretty slim, especially when the only food available is cotton candy and toxic orange nachos. I just don't get to have much fun. For all practical purposes, I simply can't stand in line for ninety minutes waiting for a ride; I would need at least two bathroom trips in that amount of time. Not to mention being locked into a ride seat that I can't escape if the dreaded moment comes.

This particular trip opened my eyes to something I didn't know about. One of the other teachers who went with us is a cancer survivor. As a result, she lost a good part of her leg in all the surgeries. She walks with a cane and a fair amount of difficulty. It turns out that most amusement parks offer a quick route into the ride for handicapped people. They have you walk up the exit path and let you in, right up front. The kids with us loved it because the parks allow a limited number of companions with each disabled person. So she spent the day ushering kids around the line so they didn't have to wait. We could debate the karma of such opportunism, but that's not my point.

What it meant to me is that such an accommodation could allow me to enjoy a place like this. But I don't have an obvious physical disability that people can recognize easily. I fear that any attempts to claim a handicap would be treated with skepticism and perhaps even resentment. Really, IBD is not the kind of disease people readily understand. They clearly see how a person in a wheelchair has difficulty with mobility. But I cringe at the thought of being seen as "someone who can't hold it," as if somehow it were a choice or a lesser challenge. Frankly, I might prefer to walk with a limp if it meant I never had to fear the humiliation of soiling myself at Six Flags and walking fifteen miles back to the car for a fresh set of clothes (if I was clever enough to have them along). Or maybe a dozen trips on the splashy log ride would do the job. Yuck.

There's another issue with amusement parks, concerts, sporting events, movies, and other controlled-access activities. All of these places will happily accommodate physical disabilities with special seating areas, wheelchair-friendly entrances, and other courtesies, but they typically have strict rules against bringing in outside food and beverages.

Digestive diseases are legitimate handicaps; though they generally are not recognized or accommodated by most places we visit.

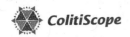

The "Americans with Disabilities Act" and other lobbying efforts have made great headway in this regard, but those of us with disabilities that receive much less attention and understanding are still left by the wayside.

The places that impose outside food restrictions typically serve mostly junk food, the sort of stuff we can not eat at all, or that give us symptomatic problems. There should be a provision in the standard ADA code if there isn't already, (and if there is it should be more widely recognized) that allows people like us to carry in our own foods. Diabetics might stand the best chance of getting leeway at the door since nearly everybody understands their issues, but many people have never heard of IBD, CD, or UC, and therefore will either be skeptical or will require copious amounts of explanation to understand. Sort of like the "Ass Pass," we should lobby for a food pass. Call it the "Gastro Pass" or something, like the handicap placard, which would make it easier (or even possible) for us to participate in these kinds of events.

Having much of our illness invisible is definitely a challenge, but on the other hand, there's the issue of when and how much we want people to know about our difficulties. As nice as it would be for others to understand that we have a significant physical challenge, sometimes we don't really want to share it with others. For example, I do a pretty good job of hiding it from my students until something relevant occurs that forces me to explain. Of course this book is likely to let the cat out of the bag, but I have faith that people will be able to handle it responsibly.

However, we need to tell some people because at times we'll need their help. But even if others know that we have this disease, they may not truly appreciate what we go through without receiving more intimate information (or something like this book!).

In any case, it's always more comforting to open up to people who you think will be understanding—which might be everybody, but when you have potentially embarrassing information about yourself, it's hard to share with just anyone. Fortunately, I have never noticed anyone react in a way that made me feel embarrassed or flawed, though that certainly is a concern for me when I breech the line of anonymity. It seems that most people are much more mature and understanding than our fears would lead us to believe. Though I have to admit that I often wonder what people are thinking after I've shared information about my condition. Do they walk away thinking that I'm somehow weak or damaged?

The other possibility, especially for close friends and family members, is that they may react with fear and denial. Most people do not enjoy being confronted with troubling news. It's natural for those around us to need some space to adjust, just as we needed time and space when we first got the news. They too must go through the stages of bewilderment, denial, anger, and fear. Some people may have trouble accepting that their child/parent/spouse/sibling/relative is having serious health problems. This is a powerful confrontation that some will have difficulty with and that may require significant effort to work through.

Remember that there are safe places to share your story with friendly ears. There are Crohn's and colitis support groups in every state, nearly all urban areas, and many other places. These wonderful resources provide places to talk openly with others who have had experiences similar to yours and who understand what you're going through. Plus, the experiences they share with you can be very enlightening, and many groups have guest speakers on relevant topics. Often support groups create their own referral network and can provide you with great information about local resources. I highly encourage you to find a support group that you can participate in.

Whatever the situation, I'm always intrigued by the reactions I get when people find out that I have IBD and learn what this means. It's not a very visible ailment, aside from what people might notice about our bathroom visits. Even those who know something is awry can be very surprised. What people often say to me after hearing about my experiences is something like, "Geez Andy, I knew you had some problems but I never knew you suffered like that," or "I had no idea you have that battle going on all the time..." and so on.

Explanations can take quite a bit of time—either because they've never heard of Crohn's or colitis or because they're very curious, or because we have a long and well-rehearsed monologue

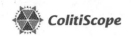

we're accustomed to performing. Usually there are questions, and then—inevitably—comes the advice.

I have found that, aside from my golf swing, nothing evokes more prolific unsolicited advice from others than having an illness. For some reason these two situations seem to invite advisory diarrhea in a form and quantity that people would otherwise never dare to offer.

"My granny always said to drink a glass of prune juice before bed."

"Have you tried yoga/hypnosis/crystals/worms?"

"My hippie sister did acupuncture to quit smoking; maybe that would help."

"You took your eye off the ball, you're rushing it, cross your wrists, it's all about follow-through, get a magnetic bracelet, yadda yadda yadda."

We've all heard comments like these, and sometimes we do learn useful information from them. The trouble is that, while we recognize people are simply trying to be helpful, it's totally natural to find it exhausting. No matter how much they want to help you, they can't control your immune system, for better or worse—but they may or may not understand that, though they truly mean well. So I try to re-characterize these comments and perceive them as being empathetic and caring rather than advisory. It is human nature for people to want to appear useful, helpful, knowledgeable, etc., but what we might need more than help, advice or information, is simple compassion.

Often what I want is for everyone else to leave it alone and let me be normal. For example, at a dinner party or family holiday, I genuinely appreciate people's efforts to accommodate or inquire about my dietary needs, but I rarely want it to be a focus of the event. I'm glad to have my needs considered, but sometimes it gets in the way when dinner discussions center on my digestive challenges, my illness, my freakdom.

And frankly, I am sure that sometimes those close to us get sick of us being the center of attention in those ways too. They tire of hearing about me and my IBD and grow weary of the inescapable repetition of these conversations. This is quite natural and perfectly reasonable. At times I have to make a conscious effort to ensure that the limelight gets shared and my issues don't dominate the conversation. Otherwise it can become a cyclic dynamic, even exhausting, on both sides.

I find it difficult to balance others' curiosity and assistance with my need to be a regular person or sometimes my need not to think about my disease just then. Maybe the conversation will remind me of an upcoming procedure or a change in medication or another juncture that I find uncomfortable—or outright frightening. Sometimes I don't want to be reminded of the fact that I'm sick, forever. These unintended internal confrontations may provoke unexpected reactions from me that the observer can't understand without knowing the complexity of my resulting thought process. That said, I also don't want to be treated like I'm fragile all the time.

I can't always tell how I'll feel or respond to people's attention. Perhaps there are situations in which I offer a response that seems to not appreciate their concern. I suppose I end up sending mixed messages. Sometimes I want to talk about it; sometimes I want to be left alone. In some cases I want my peculiarities to be accommodated, and in others I prefer to camouflage them. The only sure result of this equation for others is confusion. I admit it, though I surrender to it as well. It's confusing to me sometimes too—actually maybe a lot of the time, but I might not let you see that very often because I want to be (and appear as) a strong person. I don't always want to feel damaged, but I may often need to be cared for anyway. So my best advice for those who know me is to go with the flow. Let it be how it is that day, and know that I always appreciate their efforts, even if they don't seem to be what I need at the time.

Sometimes my family gets into a pattern in which we're all trying to out-accommodate each other. Everybody's trying to make a group decision based on what we think the others want, while assuming that any comments to the contrary are their efforts to give in and accommodate us. Then we end up with a decision that's a bizarre amalgamation of what's left over after we've eliminated what we all assume each other doesn't want. This is especially apparent when we're dining out or traveling together. There will be suggestions about museums, landmarks, sights, restaurants, and the like, but these are all assumptions about what we think the others want, or listings of alternatives to what we think each other

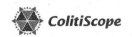
ColitiScope

would like to avoid—and then we wind up someplace truly weird, like a bowling alley.

Apply this super-accommodating approach to my health situation, and the results can be quite similar. It has been helpful to me for my friends and family to understand my disease better. However, now that I have shared a lot with them, that accommodation process tends to focus around what they think my digestive system requires, to the extent that it's hard to convince people of what I actually prefer at the time because they're so busy attending to what they assume will be helpful or what I seemed to need last time. Sometimes it's hard to convince them that my preferences for simplicity are genuine rather than polite attempts to avoid inconveniencing them.

As far as family difficulties go, this one is really not such a bad thing. A family that's so concerned with each other's comfort that it takes work to tone it down? Frankly, compared to issues I've seen friends deal with, I'd be hard pressed to even put ours in the problems category. I think we can work on that pretty easily if we trust each other to communicate honestly.

Another difficulty arises when people don't readily appreciate how important it is for me to avoid sick people. While a simple cold or flu may not be a big deal for most people, it can be devastating for me because I don't have a normal immune system. For that reason I may elect to avoid interactions with people if they're sick. It takes finesse to manage that politely without hurting feelings.

The fact that I have been relatively lucky in being able to control my disease with medication makes it a bit difficult for others to understand its seriousness. A while back I was having a discussion with a senior friend about life and death and hardship, and so on. He's sort of an old-timer from a by-gone era, so stories about the good old days abound in conversations with him. I respect him highly as a professional and as an elder who has been a mentor to me, but he sometimes forgets that he's not the only person in the room with any valid life experience.

We got to chatting about life challenges and difficulties, and I was talking about how imprisoning it can feel to know that my job is more than a mere income, it's my lifeline to health insurance. With a chronic illness, acquiring and retaining that security can be difficult, so it's a significant loss of freedom to feel tied down that way, regardless of whether I'm happy in my job or not.

"Aw, you young folks think things are so bad, but you don't realize how good you have it...I raised three kids and put them through college, *I* know what job security is all about," he said

His belittling reaction was frustrating. I raised my voice and defended myself,

"You know what, I have a chronic disease which requires medication that costs more than I make. You don't have to put three kids through college in order to have perspective on job security."

"Well I knew you had been sick, but since you don't seem to struggle with it much, I figured it wasn't that big a deal for you," he replied.

"Just because I am able to manage it well without looking miserable doesn't mean it hasn't had a profound impact on my life," I said. I'm not accustomed to talking back to him so confidently, but this time he crossed a line, and I felt the need to correct him. His response indicated that he truly is a gentleman.

"Well in that case I should apologize," he said graciously, and the conversation continued.

What this illustrates to me is that folks have a tendency to assume everything's A-OK if we don't complain a lot. It's natural for them to think we're doing fine if we don't appear to suffer—even for those who know us well and know our situation. After all, it's very tempting to focus on the good news rather than the bad in situations like this, especially when the bad is not showing itself very often.

The main challenge behind the concealed nature of our disease is that people really don't see much of it from the outside. It also involves taboo topics that people have difficulty talking about openly or inquiring about with confidence. I deal with this challenge mostly by communicating a lot. Perhaps I err on the side of telling people too much, but it is my theory that the more others know the better they will understand. Hopefully I'm right about that because I truly believe that by increasing understanding we can have the most impact on how we are treated, how the world sees our disease, and the work that gets done to research and cure it.

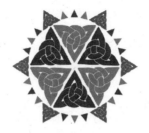

Par for the Course

Those of us living with IBD must take things as they are and try to do our best, whatever comes along. It's hard not to feel imprisoned by a disease that keeps us tied to certain places or constantly in search thereof. I am speaking of bathrooms, of course. Never has my acuity been as honed as it is now for scanning and spotting anything that looks like it is, contains, or can be converted to a toilet. I have developed a veritable porcelain radar.

At times I choose not to go places that don't seem likely to have suitable accommodations. Sometimes I just don't go out at all. When my symptoms are active, I loathe the thought of festivals, concerts, sporting events, hikes, and other situations that would leave me exposed. Fighting the urge to seek safety at all times is hard work; yet I do push myself enough to lead a somewhat normal life.

Golf courses are among the places that consistently challenge me, especially unfamiliar ones. I know my home course well and can make an efficient route to the outhouse from anywhere on it. But with new territory comes trepidation.

Last summer I went golfing with a couple of old buddies. Rick is still a close friend, but Dave is a more casual pal. Dave and I got a cart (which I often do now in case I have to make a break for it), but Rick is a die-hard purist so he insists on walking.

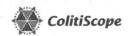

I had thoroughly inspected the course map and tried to memorize the pit stop locations throughout. However, as we got a few holes deep into the front nine, I realized that what I had thought were restrooms were actually watering holes. It is never good to discover that what you thought was your refuge turns out to be something else. Well, inevitably an issue came of it.

I am not always sure how casual friends will react to news about my illness, so I often keep it to myself until it feels safe or relevant to reveal more detail. Typically this becomes an informative discussion, which more often than I expect reveals that their lives are connected to IBD in other ways as well. Most people are interested and compassionate. Some are quite curious, which I don't mind because there are some fun stories to tell that keep it light.

In this case, Dave asked me at one point, "So, Andy, what does it mean for your daily life?" a more intuitive question than I am accustomed to fielding.

"Well, it means that I am always tied to the bathroom, always searching for one, constantly making contingency plans, and looking for an out. And sometimes it means not making it in time."

His lips opened in a sympathetic grimace revealing closed teeth behind. I could see his imagination churning, images coming to his mind, pain showing in his eyes. He audibly breathed in through his teeth.

"Yep," I inserted, nodding my head.

"Oh, dude," he said, pensively, shaking his head.

"Yep," I repeated.

As we cruised down the fairway of the next hole, I realized that I had left my sand wedge at the previous green. Rick was walking, so Dave and I had some time to go back for it in the cart. Along the way, I started to have inklings of an impending Nature 911. I discretely scanned the horizon for the clubhouse because there seemed to be no other options. Before we arrived at the abandoned wedge, I caught a glimpse of the parking lot. Victory! I made a sharp turn towards it.

"Where we goin?" Dave inquired.

"Um, remember what I just said about the bathroom? It's one of those times."

"Oh man. Well, drop me off here, and you can catch up."

I skidded the cart to a halt and let him out. Before he was even off the cart I floored it, making a bee line for you-know-where. I heard a holler behind me and turned my head to see Dave waving his arms. I understood the issue when I realized that I was peering through his golf clubs to see him—they were still mounted to my cart.

"Sorry man, I'm outta time," I shouted back to him, quickly refocusing on what had now become a baja grand prix. I approached an occupied tee box at exactly the wrong moment. Golfer etiquette generally prohibits this sort of distracting commotion. I felt a twinge of guilt for storming through while they teed off, but I reassured myself that if they knew my situation and how desperate I was, surely they'd understand. From a glance at their faces it didn't look like they did, but I gave them credit anyway.

After a jaunt through some trees, I rounded a corner with the prize in view, just 50 yards away. A moment too late, I noticed the wooden curbs laid on the ground with the painted word "Scatter." *That's exactly what I'm about to do, but hopefully inside,* I thought to myself. Unfortunately, I was going too fast and couldn't veer around the timbers. I ran over the corner of one, launching my rear wheel several inches off the ground. I landed on the seat with a dreadfully precarious impact. I had to focus for a moment to assure myself that there'd been no premature scattering. Hastily parking the cart, I quickly hobbled into the clubhouse. With great relief I barely made it in time; thank goodness there was an empty stall. Another disaster narrowly averted.

I caught up to Rick and Dave at the next tee where they were waiting for me.

"Everything come out OK?" Rick asked in a way that made me wonder if he was annoyed or just trying to be funny.

"Just-in-time delivery." I joked back. "Sorry to dump you off like that Dave, I don't get to choose the timing of these things, and I wasn't thinking about your clubs."

"That's OK Andy, I just finished the hole with your sand wedge," he said, handing it back to me. "Got a par."

Parring a hole using a single club is an impressive achievement. But in my book he deserved even better—I would have scored him a birdie for being a good sport.

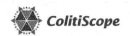

As IBD patients, we ask a lot of the people around us. We do have special needs, and our loved ones put forth significant effort and at times make sacrifices to accommodate them. I am very touched when people find ways to truly take these difficulties in stride. Patient adaptations like my wife Heather is saintly for, creative solutions like Dave's decision to go with the flow, and plain-old compassion are often the staples of my relationships now. Some of our friends and family will be naturally good at it; others will learn over time; but they will all need to adapt in some way. And at times, like us, they too will be frustrated.

Another simple story illustrates this nicely. About the time my family was starting to notice more of my daily grind, I had to make a speedy pit stop while shopping with my wife and brother. This was becoming a familiar occurrence. When I returned from the bathroom, I found they had entrenched themselves in conversation as they customarily do when I'm off in my "special place."

"It can't be normal," my brother commented, "being that urgent all the time."

"It isn't," I answered. "I have a disease."

"Yeah, but still," he said with a perplexed expression.

Yeah, it's hard to get your mind around it all sometimes; that's true for us and for our loved ones as well. We spend a lot of time learning on our own because we face the challenges constantly. But others in our lives are less confronted by them, and for that reason, they absorb the lessons at a different pace.

Family and friends experience their share of valid irritations as well. Heather waits for me, all over the place, everywhere we go. We leave late so I can use the bathroom one more time. We travel less and with more difficulty. Since we have always enjoyed adventuring together, that's a true loss for us. But lovers accommodate each other in special ways that others are not accustomed to. People around us will be affected in a variety of ways. At times our needs are absolute, and others' needs get put aside. Conversations get interrupted, plans suddenly delayed, phone calls hastily ended, car trips severely impacted.

All of our supporters will inevitably adjust, given enough time and effort. Meanwhile, we can support them with the same understanding that we expect for ourselves. While we know the people in our lives are tolerant, we can still apologize when we inconvenience or disappoint them, and we can find other ways to acknowledge the hardships we ask others to endure with us. And we can thank them, in whatever way works, to show them what their efforts mean to us.

So yes, all of this is par for the course, but it's a whole lot more fun when we enjoy the game together. That requires compassion, humor, creativity, and support—in both directions. We need a lot of it, but we can give it out too.

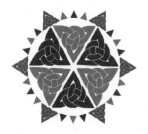

IB Dating

So, you have IBD. You're single or divorced and playing the field. Or you're in a relationship, married, or in some way romantically active or interested. Everything in the romance category boils down to one single incontrovertible truth. It's blunt, perhaps a bit crude, but we gotta get it out there, so I'm just going to say it.

It's darn-near impossible to feel sexy when you're having diarrhea every ten minutes.

Combine any IBD-related symptomatic issues and potential embarrassments you can think of with other factors such as the cosmetic side effects of medication like acne, hair loss, weight gain, stretch marks, etc., and you have the recipe for a self-esteem disaster. Plus, it's hard to get excited about intimacy when you're feeling lousy all the time.

It's tempting to shove back the realities of IBD, ignore their impact, get lazy, and lower your expectations for life. You may try to protect yourself by making romance impersonal or by avoiding intimacy altogether. This approach may work for a while, but making it last will be difficult, and it's not fair to your partner either. At first there will be adjustments, avoidance, whatever it takes to get through the initial phases of dealing with the disease. This has to be a natural part of the process. But there will need to be a transition

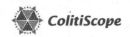

at some point, to "get back on the horse," so to speak. No matter how much we may want to retreat into ourselves and be impersonal, we have to keep it personal; indeed, that's the only way to make intimacy work.

The single most important thing to keep in mind when it comes to these issues is that our partners, if they indeed they are the loving and caring people we need them to be, *will* understand. That's hard to imagine while wrapped up in our little ball of anxiety. Our worst fears try to convince us that intimate moments will be spoiled, embarrassing, unpleasant, or simply impossible. But we don't have to listen to that catastrophic thinking. Instead, we can listen to our internal confidence, our security, our trust. The love we share with another is too big to be daunted by an occasional awkward moment. Understanding each other's needs and limitations is a part of life in all the ways we interact. If we're practiced at accommodating each other's general foibles, then we should be able to handle the more touchy issues too. In the end, it may not be as difficult as we expect.

Of course, this seems easier for people with established relationships. If you're in a new situation, that first conversation with your partner about IBD might be very intimidating. But remember that you are with this person because you want to be, and if you are truly going to enter a relationship, then you'll have to deal with the IBD issues up front together. In all likelihood, your partner will be understanding and will want to make the relationship work. Besides, remember what we're talking about here, the promise of certain rewards has a tendency to motivate! On the other hand, if your prospective partner has less aptitude for making accommodations than you need, then perhaps it's a good thing to discover that earlier rather than later. However, we need to be sure we offer them the chance (and some time) to adapt. After all, we needed an adjustment period too.

It won't necessarily be easy of course. And no matter how flexible your partner wants to be, you will both experience frustrations just as you do with other parts of your lives. The struggles with intimacy really do not have to be all that different.

I do have to admit, however, that while I'm happy to joke about it most of the time, sometimes my symptoms do make me feel gross.

After all, who really wants to feel like a liquid shit factory all the time? Obviously everything is much easier when symptoms are at bay, but for the other times we may have to call on our understanding and courage. We can't hibernate forever.

There are obvious practical issues with romance if you're on the pot every ten minutes. Even if there were time to squeeze a "quickie" in between, it might still feel uncomfortable. Plus, while ten minutes may be plenty of time for one partner, it's usually not enough for both. So get creative. Heck, if need be, just do it in the bathroom! A few candles...something cozy on the floor...whatever it takes to create a comfort zone. Plus there are lots of fun things to do without having to be fully exposed to your vulnerabilities. Find something that feels like a security blanket and figure out a way to work with it. Make it a fun adventure.

Not all of the self-image issues are logistical or physical limitations. Some are more internal. Take me for example. I used to feel fairly fit, satisfied with my self-image. But a decade or so ago, I quit smoking and gained 30 pounds in three months. That's fine, I wouldn't trade my extra weight for the incessant sinus infections and other smoking accoutrements. I got used to my belly, calling it my "workbench" (and a pretty good one), but really thinking of it as my "Quit-Smoking Trophy." And now, since my prednisone roller coaster began, another tier has been added to the trophy. It's more than a belly now. It's more like a "Superbowl Ring"; plus it also comes along with a full buffet of the aforementioned cosmetic blemishes, and a plethora of other challenges to one's self-perceived suavity. Oh joy.

I would love to change some physical characteristics to help me feel virile and attractive. I'd like to drop the gut for starters. Trouble is, the one time I tried to part with my trophy, the diet I was on conspicuously coincided with my initial colitis symptoms, and the reprise after my first remission came after a second attempt at that diet. Only in hindsight did I put the pieces together and get suspicious. So what does a person do? Obviously there are other dietary approaches, or I can accept my body for what it is. However, there are other good health benefits that come from maintaining a healthy weight, so I'm not going to give up easily.

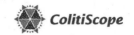

Some of the physical downsides of IBD we truly can't do anything about. The side effects of medication are generally unavoidable, though we can control them to some extent by the treatments we pursue. Prednisone is hard on a lot of people. The chubby "moon face" is a common complaint, as is weight gain. Hair loss is tough for some. My receding hairline had a head start, so I'm not sure if that's been impacted by my disease and treatment or if it's a part of my natural aging process. But I'm not overly preoccupied with it. If my hair ever starts to look bad on me, I'll just shave it off. I found the acne to be a little more interesting though; it made me feel young instead of old. When I started the steroids, suddenly I felt fifteen again. But I didn't have acne this bad as a teenager! Again, not too difficult for me, mostly it's just annoying.

But if I were a teenager now and were experiencing these things, I would certainly feel more challenged by them. I'm married; I don't have to chase girls anymore. I have established myself sufficiently in ways that give me the confidence to overcome many concerns about my appearance, so my perspective helps me now in a way that wasn't possible at a younger age. But try to tell a sixteen-year-old girl that stretch marks really aren't a big deal, and you'll quickly find out how wrong you are.

I always found the teen years to be a cruel time in life. Kids are all searching for their place in the pecking order, in the world, in the room, heck even in the car. So much rides on every little thing. There's so much pressure to be somebody, even when you're trying to be yourself, because you're not sure who that is yet. With that perspective in mind, it's easy to see what a challenge this disease presents for a young person. Then add the pressures of dating and mating into the mix, and the difficulty is multiplied.

It has been many years since I was a teenager, yet I still have scars from that time. I didn't even have IBD at that age, so I certainly sympathize with young patients. I can assure you, however, that time will bring perspective. It really is true that cosmetic issues aren't as critical as they sometimes seem, and it is healthy to accept the things we cannot change.

But there are some impacts of our disease that we can control. I am currently working on getting back to a healthy weight. I've tried a number of approaches. The one that's working for me at the moment is a scoring system that allows daily points to spend on food. I never imagined I would try a strategy like this, but it's actually a sensible approach. It's not about deprival but about learning how to make smarter decisions for yourself. The numerical strategy conjures up baggage from my upbringing that should make me reject it on principle (my father had a point system for absolutely everything), so I hate to admit this, but it is actually quite effective for me.

There are a zillion ways to approach the weight-management challenge. I'd be careful to avoid the shocker diets or others that require dramatic menu changes. I've learned from experience how traumatic those can be on my system. So now I take an easy-does-it approach and try to focus on making good choices. That seems to be working for me.

Instead of only dwelling on physical attributes we'd like to change, it is also useful to work on expanding and improving our repertoire of coping skills. Accepting ourselves for who we are seems like such a simple concept when people say it, but really it's not so easy. How do you do that exactly? Learning to be confident and feel good about yourself can be an elusive process. There are a lot of skills to use and develop. There are plenty of self-help books with ideas to try for yourself. Don't be afraid to seek a therapist for help if you would like some guidance. There's nothing to be ashamed of. After all, we hire all sorts of professionals to help us in many ways, so why not do the same for this critical objective? There are volumes of resources available and many people who can help on this topic, so try some of them and see what works best for you.

We need to make peace with our disease. It may often feel like an unwanted foreign entity that should be rejected and repelled, but that simply isn't going to happen. Instead we must learn to own it, to integrate it into our lives, and to embrace it as a part of ourselves. This may require significant effort and introspection. We may need to employ outside resources. And we may never finish. This is more a process than a destination, and it will likely evolve over time. Hopefully, we will find peace along the way.

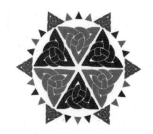

Diet Schmiet

If you're like most patients, I would guess that you have heard doctors say things similar to what I heard from mine about diet—that food has nothing to do with IBD—it is not caused by dietary issues, and they don't even advise avoiding spicy foods anymore. "That was an old wives tale," they claim. Interesting how docs can say such things so confidently when they seem to have absolutely no idea what does cause IBD. Regardless of what the M.D.s say about it, ask any Crohn's or colitis patient if their symptoms are related to their diet and you get an emphatic, unanimous YES. Absolutely!

Now before we conclude that medical professionals are completely oblivious to the diet-symptom relationship, it might be helpful to take a quick look from their perspective. They work in an environment where scientific studies call the shots. Any solid conclusions must be based on established proof, which generally comes from double-blind, placebo-controlled studies in which statistics are carefully analyzed to generate decisive numerical results. That approach seems straightforward enough when applied to drug testing, but think about it as a test for dietary factors. I am certainly stumped by how one might develop a placebo for spicy food. It seems to me that in an effort to provide us only with verifiable information, doctors sometimes decline to provide potentially helpful advice unless it has been scientifically proven. This doesn't mean they're wrong, but it does suggest they're probably not our best resource for this kind of information.

So with or without the doctor's help, how do you discover a reasonable diet that works compatibly with your digestive disease? It's an incredibly personal thing. I have no problem with spicy foods, but nuts really mess me up. I've tried eliminating various categories of foods. Some individual foods seem to make a lot of trouble for me so I avoid those too. Romaine lettuce, for example, is not good for me. All other kinds of lettuce seem to be OK, but romaine basically works like intestinal floss—and in a big hurry. I don't understand the origins of all these variables, but I do learn what I can and cannot eat. And for each person these things will differ greatly—there is no universal solution.

Eating in a restaurant can be a real challenge. Sometimes I just can't bring myself to do it. Partly it's the bathroom thing (for which take-out has become my favored solution), but there's also the mystery factor. Sure the menu and staff can help you try to understand what you're ordering, but you can never anticipate exactly what all the ingredients will be in restaurant food. It takes time to experiment with a menu to find out what you can tolerate. Then it's good to stick with what you know. That's one way I can eat out relatively safely, though that's assuming the preparation will be consistent, which is not always the case. But I have to avoid some places all together.

One particular fast food taco shack is consistently bad for me, so I stay away (I won't mention the name, but I'm sure you'd know it). Their food is a guaranteed laxative in my system. "Laxplositive" is more like it. Sure, most fast food is junk food, but it doesn't all affect me in the special way the food in this place does. Along with my meal, I receive a guaranteed toilet grenade within five minutes—every time. The only way I can imagine eating that stuff is if I were already sitting on the toilet.

If you experience something similar (which many do as it is common even for people without digestive illnesses), I'll let you in on a little secret that can save you lots of aggravation. Get your order for take-out, bring it home, and take it into the bathroom. Before you sit down, unwrap the tacos and just throw them straight into the toilet. It's the best approach as far as I can tell. The results are pretty much the same as if you'd eaten them, only you spare yourself the pain and save some toilet paper, and it's a low-fat solution as well. How's that for a weight-loss program?

I have an affinity for certain foods my wife finds so vile that she won't even come near them. She makes a guttural gagging sound whenever they're mentioned—barbeque and sloppy joes seem to conjure the more pronounced responses from her. It seems that, in just about any digestive state, I can tolerate certain foods that others find questionable. But when I'm flared up, everything comes out in a hurry, so I don't notice their individual impacts very much. For most of us, certain foods provoke more digestive trauma than others, which is why it's important to take a disciplined approach to tracking that information. I have heard from so many people that keeping a food diary is a lifesaver: tracking what they eat, how they process the food, and how it makes them feel. Some even document their emotional state and find useful correlations.

I have tried a number of programmatic approaches. One book I read claimed that many IBD sufferers find relief by eliminating fructose from their diet. Fructose is a sweetener made from corn syrup. I decided to give it a try. I started buying foods that were sweetened with cane sugar instead. Then I started trying to eliminate fructose from other sources as well and made a startling discovery. It's nearly impossible to find foods that aren't loaded with the stuff. Bread, crackers, meat products, TV dinners—all sorts of packaged foods that shouldn't be sweet are fructose filled. It's amazing, the stuff is everywhere. Even in fruit juice! That seems especially crazy because most natural food items use fruit juices for sweeteners as alternatives to sugar—but look at the bottled fruit juices in the grocery store and you'll find they have extra sugar added in the form of fructose. The ones that claim to have no sugar added instead have artificial sweeteners like sucralose or aspartame. Even naturally sweet foods are "enhanced" with these insidious products.

Everything that doesn't need sugar has it, and everything that already has sugar gets more. Considering all that caloric surplus being ingested unnecessarily, it's no wonder our population has so many health problems related to excess weight. I know the food industry is just trying to make us like their products, but if they kill off their customer base, they won't have anyone to sell them to.

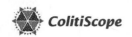

Foresight doesn't seem to be an American virtue anymore, at least not when there's money to be made on ignoring it.

In any case, the fructose elimination diet didn't do much for me. I did cut out dairy products permanently, and that helped a lot. Funny, I never realized how much aggravation dairy foods were causing me until I stopped ingesting them. Suddenly my prolific gas factory shut down. That was a good thing—trust me or just ask Heather!

I am currently experimenting with a low-gluten diet. I've never been diagnosed with celiac disease, which is gluten intolerance, but I have found that when I eat carbs in other forms, my system is much happier, and stools are mostly solid even when I do have inflammation. I'm pretty well convinced that I am better off without gluten, but I'm not super-diligent about it. I've mostly eliminated the major sources of wheat products, such as bread and pasta, so tragically, there goes my third true love, mac and cheese.

Funny how people often say things like "I couldn't live without X" or "I'd die if I couldn't have Y." These are statements made by people in good health. They remind me of people who have never had back problems but claim chiropractors are quacks. When presented with miserable symptoms, especially frightening or embarrassing ones, people learn quite quickly that they can do without many foods (or other comforts), even ones they love.

I have also tried dietary approaches geared toward my particular blood type—mine is called the "caveman diet," which means I get to eat a lot of meat. It sounds so manly I almost find it worthwhile for that reason alone. It also works pretty well, however, so bring it on!

With so many avenues to explore, I could spend a lot of time sorting out all the options. At the very least, paying more attention to what I eat has made me think more about what a healthy diet means and how to achieve it. A professional would be a great help to me I am sure, which is why I appreciated the dietician who made a presentation to my Crohn's and colitis support group.

I was never an apt pupil for biology, so I must say that I'm suffering significant knowledge gaps when it comes to my body, what kind of nourishment it needs, and in what foods to find it. As a human being, it's probably one of the worst things to be ignorant about. Yet here I am doggie-paddling through a sea of nutritional mystery. I definitely could use a coach, at least to learn some basics and skills. And my wife is in the same boat. One of her colleagues, a biology teacher, got a chuckle once when Heather thought that amino acids were something you'd find in a chemistry set.

But regardless of what the books and the scientists say, it's important to pay attention to what your body tells you. After discovering that my body does better on rice than wheat, I finally understood why I always crave Asian food. Certain foods always generate perfect stool for me. I have fewer digestive issues the more meat I eat. These kinds of subtle indicators may be the best advice available, and they're absolutely custom tailored to each person, so be sure to listen for them and act upon them as well.

Gaining an understanding of the foods that are good for me and the ones I should avoid has become a process rather than a program. It's an ongoing experiment with a single subject—me—and new data every day. As I develop my own system, I realize that its up to me to formulate my own conclusions and to honor the actions they suggest. This is a crucial step toward a managed IBD lifestyle, and it varies so much with each person that specific advice can not be universally applied. In addition, your condition will likely evolve over time, so your diet will need to adapt accordingly. There is no easy or consistent answer.

Be especially wary of those who suggest miracle diets and web sites with cult followings. These may be successful approaches for some people, maybe even a lot of people, but not necessarily for you. What works for someone else, or even for a lot of people, may or may not affect you positively and could have a negative impact.

What we certainly can't do is make medical judgments about our own disease based on our response to what foods do or do not work for others. These details are far too individualized to be applied in a general sense. We should use caution in how we treat information we get from others. Everyone wants to be helpful. But for better or worse, we must each determine what dietary regimen works best for us. We need to do that based on our own experience.

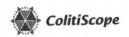

ColitiScope

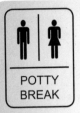

POTTY BREAK

Eating and food issues are always topics for adventure. Once, in the bathroom of a Thai Restaurant, I was sitting in the stall when a little kid, maybe eight or nine years old, came in and looked around. I guess he needed a number two because he ignored the urinal and peered in at me through the crack. He stepped back after a couple seconds, and just before leaving the room he stopped and said, "Pee-eew mister, you stink!"

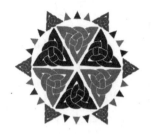

Immunosuppressed

So how fragile am I? I read the warnings on my medications, all of which suggest that I will be prone to infections and illness because the meds compromise my immune system. Well, what exactly is meant by "use caution?" It is easy to get the impression from all the warnings that I should live in a bubble. Should I avoid hospitals? Foreigners? Certain places, people, or events? I figure that, at the very least, I should stay away from sick people. OK, I get that, but easier said than done.

I work at a university. College kids get everything and not only spread local bugs around campus but bring germs back from all over the place—home, spring break, their Habitat for Humanity project in New Guinea. How am I supposed to keep my distance when I'm working with them all the time? And that's just my half of the equation. My wife is a high school teacher. She spends her whole day in a Petri dish, incubating a buffet of germs from thousands of kids. Ever look at the epidemiology studies and government reports on preparations for outbreaks? Ever notice how teachers are the first to die in the damage forecasts? The first thing all those response plans suggest is to close the schools. Great, I'm on the front line of the germ defense echelon. And it's not just myself, my wife is a conduit as well, though her immune system seems to be steel-clad, so that's a plus, as long as she doesn't carry it all back to me.

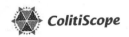

I may tend toward being unnecessarily anxious about certain things, but some of them carry real risks. I am left wondering how to make sense of it all. I want to be prudent but not paranoid. This balance is an elusive prize. Do I really get sick more easily while on these medications? If I get sick, will I get better? Will it provoke my IBD symptoms? If I have to take antibiotics will my colitis flare up again? How much caution is enough? Too little? Too much? I go through this emotional battle every time I have an inkling that I may be getting sick. One of the reasons I fear contagious illnesses so much is the memory of that particularly nasty sinus infection, when I took antibiotics that sent my colitis into its worst flare ever, landing me at the Mayo Clinic for a week. So not only might I be extra-susceptible to infection, I can't just pop the "cillin-du-jour" pills like regular people.

It's certainly tempting to resent the medications I take for introducing this immunosuppressant vulnerability. It's only natural to feel the irony of medicine that makes me both well and sick.

Prednisone is problematic in so many ways. Yeah, this is the stuff to get if you want to feel crazy, sweat profusely, get fat, zitty and depressed, and break your hip at forty. But look at the bright side, it can really work miracles—I started taking it, and suddenly I could eat chili dogs in the car. It seems as though all illnesses have treatments that bring both good and bad results. This fact is one of the driving forces behind the natural medicine movement. We all sometimes have to weigh options and make difficult choices. Whether my meds make me more vulnerable or not, I'd still rather not be bleeding out the rear end, so I put up with the ugly stuff.

I sit here writing this the day after an urgent warning was issued at work about a gastroenteritis outbreak. Apparently kids were barfing themselves silly all over campus. The health department set up shop; inspectors converged upon the cafeteria; and those of us responsible for teaching facilities were asked to sanitize surfaces that students come in contact with. Of course, this came on a Thursday, my maximum exposure day. I teach labs all day long, fiddling with computers and electronic equipment that students have been touching and sneezing on all day.

So we sent somebody to the store for a half-gallon mega-jug of hand sanitizer and a tub of disinfectant wipes. The store only had two tubs left, so I suppose everyone had the same idea. I gathered an army of student workers and set them to work scouring the desks, counters, workbenches, doorknobs, light switches, and the equipment: oscilloscopes and signal generators, power supplies, keyboards, and mice. I must say, some of that stuff was overdue for a cleaning anyway, and the whole facility now has a lemon fresh scent.

I walked around all day with the hand sanitizer, goofily (but only half-joking), dispensing it to anyone who would hold out a hand. I made it into a comical adventure. Perhaps that helped to ease the students' nerves about the issue, and it also cleverly disguised my outright horror. I would have been happy to coat the entire room with the stuff. I was nervous all day. Could I avoid contracting the bug? Had I gotten it already? On the way to work that morning, I had to exit at the wildlife refuge visitor center for an emergency pit stop (I had to go there because the nearby rest area is getting new bathrooms built; it's been closed for several months while two guys lay about one brick a day). My system has been fairly stable lately, so I wonder if that pit stop was a fluke or a precursor to puke. I washed my hands obsessively and used a lot of pumps from the sanitizer jug. This morning I don't feel great, but I don't have my head in the toilet either, so my fingers are still crossed.

It doesn't always take an event like this to get my anxious response going. Every time I feel any stomach distress I immediately worry if my colitis symptoms are returning. My imagination quickly leads me into a worried state. It can be difficult to stay calm during these uncertain periods. It's not unusual for a person to have digestive distress periodically, but I can't assume the symptoms are routine. Instead I end up waiting nervously until they go away. Unfortunately, in some cases, more dreaded symptoms appear, and I am faced with a colitis flare-up, which is always a depressing situation.

Events like these are the more obvious anxiety provokers. But there's a daily onslaught of other possible sources of illness. First of all, others around us are not necessarily as cautious as we are. They don't suffer the same potential repercussions from getting sick that I do, so I am aware that I have to hold a higher standard to compensate (and Heather has graciously adapted her routines to

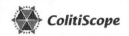

accommodate as well). But I'm also vigilant in other ways. I handle meat with extreme caution. I watch others prepare my food. I don't share utensils or drinking vessels with anyone. And I do take care to avoid places that are likely to have concentrations of germs, or at the very least I take extra precautions to protect myself. I open the bathroom door with the used paper towel; I don't touch anything at the hospital. I never put my fingers in or near my nose, mouth or eyes unless I've just washed them. I wear a surgeon's mask on the airplane even though it makes me look stupid. Antibacterial soap and hand sanitizer are my staples. My life sometimes seems to be what transpires in staccato intervals between hand-washings.

Still, despite my precautions, there are situations that take me by surprise. I served on the judging staff for the International Science and Engineering Fair when it was in town last year. It was an incredible experience. Brilliant kids brought amazing projects from all over the globe. But what I hadn't considered, despite my hyper-vigilant sense of caution, was that kids from all over the world bring germs from all over the world. And not everyplace immunizes their children against the common illnesses that we're accustomed to feeling protected from. So when word got out that there had been a measles case at the fair, and people were being urged to exercise caution and be aware of possible symptoms, I couldn't help but wonder how my paranoia could have failed to anticipate that possibility. I'm usually pretty good at dreaming up things to worry about; how could I have missed something so obvious? I'm glad I didn't think of it earlier though, because I'm sure I enjoyed the event more than I would have with that concern in my head.

I didn't give the measles case a lot of thought, however, until ten days later when I developed a mild case of tonsillitis. I did some web research on tonsillitis to see what I could learn and discovered that measles is among the most common causes. I went back and read the warnings from the science fair. "Symptoms begin to appear approximately ten days after exposure." Their advice was to check your immunization status and if it's negative or unclear to get immunized immediately.

I didn't know for sure if I'd been immunized for measles. I knew I couldn't go get vaccinated though, because the Mumps/Measles/Rubella inoculation is a live vaccine. People with compromised immune systems are advised against receiving it because they might actually contract the illness as a result.

The previous summer, a campus bulletin had been issued about kids possibly bringing measles back to school, urging us to get an immunity test or simply to be immunized. So I took the test. The results took a while to come back, and I only got a casual notice from the campus health office. I didn't worry much about it at the time because by then the students had returned and the feared outbreak did not come to fruition. So I didn't remember what the test concluded. But now with the new warnings, I wished I had paid more attention. To complicate matters slightly, that day I was packing for a trip to Colorado with friends, one of whom was eight months pregnant, so I didn't want to be responsible for spreading measles to a new community and possibly an unborn child.

I called the campus health center. They had some trouble finding a record of my visit. I'm not a student, so my case was outside their normal routine. I urged them to look again, but they couldn't find my results. As the day progressed, my tonsillitis seemed to be worsening, so I decided to call the health department phone number advertised by the science fair. I didn't know what to expect, but I've seen movies—a small part of me wondered if they'd show up at my house in a black van and haul me away. At the very least I was expecting a bureaucratic hassle.

Quite to my surprise, however, the health department was very easy to deal with. A call screener asked me a number of questions, the answers to which were apparently compelling enough to get me transferred to a doctor. He was very interested in my symptoms and my activities at the fair, and I was quite interested in knowing if I should travel or not. He mentioned that so far I was the first respondent to display the full set of warning signs and told me that they needed to do some checking. About fifteen minutes later I received a call from the supervising physician. He clarified a few details with me and quickly concluded they would need a solid confirmation of my immunization status. I explained about the test I'd taken months back and that I had trouble getting the results. He seemed to think he could locate them, so he asked for my social security number and said he'd call back. I also provided my fax number so he could

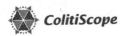

ColitiScope

forward the results to me. I hung up and prepared myself for an afternoon of the run-around.

Instead the fax machine rang about four minutes later. Out rolled a copy of my test results. Apparently, when the state health department needs information, they can get it! Of course it was written in some sort of techno-speak I couldn't comprehend, so I was glad to hear the phone ring. It was the physician calling. The test concluded that I was indeed immune to the measles, and I had nothing to worry about. He gave me emphatic clearance to go ahead with the planned vacation, and so I did.

Living with hyper-vigilance like this can be a roller coaster. Some people are paranoid about getting sick; some don't worry about that sort of stuff. Others may think we're crazy for worrying about it so much, but most people have less at stake then we do. They can afford to be more casual about it. I concern myself with the immunosuppression to a healthy degree for me. I take precautions, but don't allow the fears to cripple me in an obsessive way. As a result, in the four years since my last major flare-up, I have had only one cold and one flu (which came two days after getting a flu shot, making me hesitant to do that again). That's really amazing for me. I used to have at least three or four colds a year, and about half of those turned into sinus infections. My new regime seems to protect me from that, despite the immunosuppressant medications.

My routine is centered on three fundamental components. First, I wash and sanitize my hands regularly and keep them out of my mouth, nose, and eyes. Second, I avoid exposure to sick people and avoid contact with germs whenever possible (shake hands only when necessary, touch as few contaminated surfaces as possible, etc.). Finally, and this I believe to be the most important element, I irrigate my sinuses daily. This does wonders for me. It may seem strange and uncomfortable but it's not bad at all. The old-fashioned Netti pot is still commonly available, but it's fairly useless—gravity can't do the job by itself. It takes the Neil-Med sinus rinse bottle to do it right. This is a squeeze bottle that forces the solution through your sinuses, flushing out the gunk and keeping the nasal tissues moist. I do the rinsing process in the shower, toward the end after my sinuses have been loosened up by the steam. The rinse kit comes with saline packets that you pour into the bottle of distilled water, which you can warm in the microwave. I don't understand why this is so effective, but since I started irrigating regularly, I have not had a single sinus infection (when normally I would have had at least a half dozen). It seems to me that the saline solution flushes out the incubating junk that would otherwise fester and make me sick. That may be old-wives-tale thinking, but I don't care. It works for me; my evidence supports it, and so I believe it.

While I never would have expected to be sick less than ever while on medications that suppress my immune system, it has turned out that way. Though it's not without effort, or at times, anxiety. Does all my vigilance pay off? I don't know for sure, but it certainly seems worthwhile. Either way, I wouldn't be a believer if it weren't so effective.

Damaged Goods / Death of a Dream

Those Six Dirty Words: "For the Rest of Your Life"

During the early stages of my IBD treatment, I became aware that it would involve a lot of medications. Eventually, I even came to realize that I had a chronic illness that I would likely need to battle over the long term. But it struck me in an especially depressing way when my doctor finally said flat out, "Andrew, you're going to be on medication for this for the rest of your life."

It doesn't seem like that statement should be so shocking. But it echoed deep in the complex emotional support structure I was building up under my illness. I've tried a lot of medications; some have worked to varying degrees; others not at all. The only drug that really seems to work with regularity is prednisone, which, of course, I can't stay on forever. The long-term side effects can be devastating to the body. If it turns out that I have ulcerative colitis and not Crohn's disease, I really hope safer treatments are developed or that I get a colectomy, before I destroy my body with medication.

To this point, my meds have been relatively manageable in cost and scope. But lately we've been talking about making some more significant changes to my medication protocol.

Remicade is now coming to the front of our list of possibilities. My doctor is pushing for it. I am resisting it. Sure, I don't like starting new meds. I read all the warnings and get paranoid. I realize that I've been pretty lucky with my response to other drugs so far, aside from the miserable craziness of steroids.

But moving up to Remicade seems like a big step. First, it's a different kind of immune system modifier. They call it a "biologic," and it targets a particular agent called Tumor Necrosis Factor (TNF). Having no previous experience with this kind of medication, I have no idea how I will respond to it. Second, it has a small, but not dismissible, chance of causing allergic reactions that can be mild or life threatening in some cases. Some patients' bodies reject it, which can happen immediately, after several treatments, or upon restarting the drug after a recess. Third, it has a whole new set of possible side effects and complications. Among those are the possibilities of activating dormant tuberculosis and causing some nasty cancers. Fourth, it is an infusion administered intravenously over a several-hour period. To me, infusions that last for several hours are in a whole new league, and this new set of potential problems is worrisome.

A visit to the infusion center eased my nerves to some extent. I explained my situation and concerns, and the head nurse was kind enough to show me around the facility, so I could see what to expect from the treatments. She did a good job of addressing my barrage of questions. I was reassured by it all but still not eager to jump right in. Later I started researching the costs. Holy mackerel, the quotes I got were outrageous. I have good insurance, which pays pretty well, but I couldn't believe my ears when I heard the news.

Six weeks worth of Remicade would cost twelve thousand dollars! That's two thousand per week, two hundred eighty-five bucks a day. I would be spending about twelve dollars per hour, twenty-four hours a day. That's twenty cents per minute. But look at the bright side: hour-for-hour, it's cheaper than going to the movies. At that level of expense, why don't I just get the colectomy? It would only cost as much as a treatment or two. Trouble is that if it turns out I have Crohn's after all, I'd be in the same boat as before but now missing an organ. Oh yeah, and surgery has its dangers too!

I checked with some familiar clinic locations in other cities, and they quoted about half what my local hospital charges for Remicade. Surprisingly, the drug is the primary expense; in fact it's so expensive that it makes the associated lab and infusion fees look insignificant by comparison. I then consulted with my employer's benefits advisor and the insurance company to see if they would be interested in saving money by flying me to one of these other locations for treatments. Not surprisingly, yet also incredibly, they said no. Even though it would save them six thousand dollars every six weeks, they wouldn't buy me a plane ticket. Whatever.

Humira might be another option. It is a closely related drug with a slightly different formulation (its made entirely of human proteins, while Remicade comprises a mix of human and mouse proteins). Humira is administered by injection, however, so it's much simpler to use. I have heard conflicting reports of its cost, but it's in the same general league as Remicade. It also has a similar story regarding complications, and it has a shorter track record, so it's not exactly an easy substitute.

News like this makes a person think about what they're worth. Not as a value, but as an expense. I can't help but feel like a burden in light of these costs. With all the statistics about the rising price of health care and about how the few who draw large expenses make it more expensive for everyone, it's hard to feel good about a dose of medication that costs more than surgery. Something's definitely fishy.

But this ironic dilemma is nothing new. We've become accustomed to insane paradoxes in our economy. I can go to the store and buy a microwave oven for forty bucks—complete with complex electronics, motors, lights, and a spinning turntable, for crying out loud. Or for the same price, I can get a clear plastic skin for my iPod (which costs less to manufacture than the cardboard box the microwave comes in). Why should we expect anything different from our health care commerce?

Despite how I may need the medicine, despite how priceless I may consider life to be, despite how I'd come up with the money somehow on my own if needed to save my life, feeling like a financial burden to society really sucks. I don't want to be one of those who drain the system. It leaves me feeling broken and expensive.

My sister-in-law is trying to make me fall in love with Alaska. I have been reading a book she gave me that tells the story of a fifty-something guy who decided to isolate himself in the Yukon bush and build a log cabin to live in by himself. He brought his clothes, a few hand tools, a gun, and a can of sourdough starter. And he succeeded. What a cool thing to do; it sounds completely idyllic.

In one form or another we've all fantasized about such independence, autonomy, and self-reliance. We've all daydreamed about being stranded on a tropical island, faced with creating our own solitary civilization, living off the fruits of land and sea. But when I engage in these fantasies, it's no longer as much fun. Nowadays I lament that such an adventure is not possible for me. Without my medications, I won't make it. I can't be self sufficient. I am tethered to civilization. This human is not capable of autonomy. I am the person who has to be let back into my home for prescription meds during a forest-fire evacuation. I am the one who will die first in the dystopian post-apocalypse story. I will not be the strong survivor who rings in the new era.

The audacity of the human spirit tempts us all to feel like we could be that lone wolf, but the defect of my human body ensures that I never would. Coming to a realization like this is a deflating crossroad in life.

My capabilities for lone heroics also took another hit recently. I tried to give blood last week. I have never been terribly squeamish about blood, but I could never get myself to let a large quantity of it leave me—to voluntarily watch it drain into a bag. However, there was a blood drive on campus, and one of my students made a personal request that I consider donating. Interesting how something as simple as asking can be so effective a motivator.

I gave it some thought and concluded that I really had nothing to fear. Heck, they take my blood every time I go in for a procto exam, so I shouldn't have any trouble donating blood. It would just take a little longer. Besides, the lab techs are always drooling over my engorged veins; occasionally they'll tell me flat out that I should be a donor. My only true hesitation was whether any of the medications I take would preclude me from donating blood. I did some online research and found that there's a relatively short list of such exclusions. So I figured I'd go and see. I headed over to the gym and managed to recruit a familiar student along the way.

I checked in and was immediately taken to a booth for the safety screening. The first inquiry was whether I wanted to donate whole blood or only platelets, which would require processing my blood and returning it to my body.

"No way!" I said, "If you want my blood, you can take it and keep it, but you're not putting it back inside me after running it through a machine." She laughed. That was more than I was up for on my first try.

After a bunch of questions about overseas travel and lifestyle inquiries, we finally landed on a stumbling block. The nurse was not familiar with IBD. My colitis is indeterminate, so I explained that I might have Crohn's or ulcerative colitis and that nobody was totally sure. She disappeared for a moment and returned with the bad news. Crohn's Disease is what they call a "permanent deferral," which means not only do I not get to donate blood today, but they also logged me in the computer, so I can never "accidentally" give blood in the future without sending up warning flags. Colitis would have been OK, she said, but not Crohn's.

Wow, what a downer. The one way in which pretty much everyone is promised they can be a hero is now out of my reach. I would never want my blood to damage someone, but the fact that I was forever excluded from donating blood is a vivid reminder of my permanent flaw. I had recruited someone to donate, so in the end I felt like I had at least contributed something to the blood drive effort. (Thank you, David, for saving a life on my behalf.)

I don't know why they exclude Crohn's patients. Perhaps it's due to the mystery of our disease; maybe it's something about our meds or genes. But I am not too preoccupied with that. What really concerns me is that I intend to be an organ donor. Will this preclude me from sharing my organs when the time comes? I certainly hope not. I still have spectacularly good eyesight (perhaps that's one of my consolations for enduring digestive hardships), so it seems that at least someone should get my miracle eyes. If I were excluded

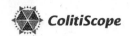

from donating my organs, it would feel tragic—to know that my body is completely useless to anyone else, even the recyclers, and that my lifesaving parts would go to waste.

The key issue is not merely feeling like damaged goods. This is about losing a fundamental human birthright: The impression built into each of us that suggests we could be the hero or go it alone if need be. That if we were willing to take life by the horns, we could live in the wild or cross a mountain range unassisted—or that we could save another's life with our own.

I believe these daydreams we indulge are an essential part of the human psyche. We all need to feel virile, capable, and self-reliant. But when certainty arrives insisting otherwise, that ideal we uphold comes crashing down. It may seem silly to mourn the loss of something that so few actually achieve in real life, but that's not the point. The important part is that we know deep down such independence is available to us if we choose to pursue it, and it makes us feel alive. So when that is freedom is taken away, it is a true loss, whether we would have engaged the pursuit or not. Knowing that we can't is the death of a dream.

Ten Universal Bathroom Truths

An open letter to architects, business owners, custodians, and building code authors

A teacher at heart, I make a concerted effort to impart a sense of perspective to my engineering students—to help them understand the needs and mindset of the end user of the products they will design and to incorporate these insights into the design process. Sitting in my office one day after a frustrating bathroom visit, I got to wondering why better bathroom designs aren't more common.

It seems clear to me that restrooms and the associated maintenance and supplies are treated like unwanted compulsory additions to a building. All too often they are designed to meet only the minimum legal criteria at the lowest possible cost. Creating a barely-legal facility might keep somebody out of jail, but it shouldn't win any awards. If the slightest bit of thought were put into how much time each person spends in the can and if that time were added up for all the people who will use the facility over the lifespan of the building, there would emerge a compelling constituency to take seriously.

These design compromises are common in both residential and commercial contexts. Bathrooms rarely stay in their originally designed form for very long, however, so it's not all the architect's fault. Remodels cheat the bathroom to maximize space elsewhere. New vendor contracts result in new dispensers. Building codes and other issues force alterations—many of which get implemented after the fact by someone who may or may not have the benefit of training or insight into the human factors of industrial design. Or the changes are handed down by frugal money handlers who either don't consider or don't care about how the changes will impact people. Often it seems like the design or alteration was performed by someone who has never used a toilet before!

Those of us with IBD and other digestive ailments use bathrooms more than any other group I suspect. Couldn't we, as power-users, be able to influence the way these facilities are designed, updated, and equipped? I certainly hope so. Therefore I feel compelled to take advantage of this opportunity to have some impact. In case this book ever falls into the hands of someone in a position to act on it with influence, I ask you to please pay attention to this chapter. It's my new *Bathroom Ergonomics 101* text.

The upcoming list is a set of observations, demands, pet peeves, requests, directives, etc. Whatever name you put on it, this is a collection of issues that are too commonly overlooked or ignored and definitely need some attention. If you are also frustrated by these concerns then please, by all means, lobby for change—at whatever level you can. Start locally and work out from there. Here's my advice to those in charge.

1. Stall doors should never swing inward unless they truly allow enough space to stand comfortably in the stall while the door closes. Apparently in an effort to avoid the *occasional* possibility of the door colliding with a passer-by, all users must suffer the cumbersome hassle of pinching themselves inside a tiny stall in order to shut the door *every time*. Basically, it's a solution that creates a bigger problem than the one it prevents. It's bad enough in most restrooms, but nowhere is this more evident than at an airport where they try to make you believe that you'll accidentally trigger Armageddon if you lose sight of your bags. It's utterly impossible to enter a bathroom stall with a suitcase unless you're wearing it on your head, and even then it would be a challenge.

2. At least one stall needs to have a sink in it. I have heard from many ostomy patients (who have had surgery that requires their stool to be collected in an external reservoir) how this would make their lives so much easier—to be able to deal with their apparatus properly in the privacy of a stall. This would be great for the rest of us too for that occasional accident or messy cleanup.

3. Trash receptacles need to be in the right places and easy to use. Put a trash can next to the exterior door, or you'll eternally be finding towels on the floor near the doorway. Refuse containers should not need to be touched to operate; preferably don't use any kind of lid. Spring-loaded closures and other blockades get what they deserve—trash on the floor. Finally, if they're not included in all the stalls, then at least the handicap stall needs a garbage receptacle. Women are not the only ones who generate non-flushable refuse.

4. Hot-air hand dryers are worthless. Yes worthless, and don't let anyone convince you otherwise, for any reason. Definitely don't install the new turbo-jets unless you want to get sued for hearing damage—either that or be prepared to hand out free earplugs to people as they enter. The first rule of air dryers is *Wipe hands on pants*. Hand towels have other important purposes in the can besides drying hands, so you gotta have them (toilet paper makes a poor washcloth, sanitary door opening requires a towel, etc).

5. If you're going to have some touch-free appliances in the room, then they have to actually work, and users shouldn't be forced to touch anything after using them. Ever feel like you're conducting an orchestra trying to coax water out of an automatic faucet? Does anybody really think it's more sanitary to use a touch-free sink valve if you have to hand-crank the towel dispenser afterwards or open the door with your hand? Few things irritate me more than an unnecessary interface with a crank, handle, lever, etc. Most of these could be prevented by having exit doors swing out, so they don't need to be touched, or by putting a toe pull at the bottom of the door.

6. If there are piles of paper scraps on the floor under your TP dispensers it means they suck, or your TP is too thin, or both. Yes, it's a miracle of modern technology that manufacturers can make toilet paper exactly one atom thick, but that doesn't mean it's a good idea. And it certainly doesn't mean you should buy it. Also, please don't try to ration the TP by some mechanical means; people will get as much as they need one way or another, so why make it harder than it needs to be? A convention I attended in Miami comes to mind. On a hot and humid Memorial Day weekend, I sat in a bathroom with a boiler room next door. It was a hundred degrees and ninety percent humidity. Sweat was virtually spurting from my pores like little geysers. Lacking the tensile strength to turn the humongous roll, the nearly-transparent toilet paper pulled off in tiny pieces that dissolved into my sweaty hands like cotton candy. Utterly useless. This is far too common.

7. Nobody takes a crap while lying on the floor, so don't install your huge donut roll dispenser at a height where it can only be reached by lying on the floor. Raise it up where you can actually reach inside it. Or better yet, don't use the huge donut at all; buck up and buy the real stuff in normal size rolls. Furthermore, caged toilet paper sucks—if you're going to provide paper, then put it out there where it can be used.

8. If you use crappy toilet paper and/or dispensers in your place of business, you are making a statement. You are telling your customers that you don't want their business and telling your employees that their comfort and practical needs are your lowest priority.

9. Low flow toilets don't work. Blah, blah, save water, cry me a river, they DON'T WORK, and they certainly don't save water when it takes several flushes to do the job! Maybe they work well in laboratory tests, thus proving to regulators and procurement officers that they're better than the old fashioned kind—but in the real world, after installation, normal use, and aging, they simply do not perform. They're much like those engineered wood products that sponge into uselessness the first time they get wet, which is usually several months before the construction project is even finished.

10. In dry climates where evaporation occurs quickly, water needs to be poured into the floor drain regularly so the sewer doesn't stink up the place. Just like under a sink, there's an odor trap in the floor drain, use it. No, don't prop the door open instead; that just stinks up the hallway.

11. Bonus! Personal preferences that should be universal: These ideas might not be universally accepted, so this honorary eleventh category isn't really in the top ten, but it's worth including.

• *A toilet seat is an adjustable appliance.* Therefore all users should be responsible for adjusting it to their own needs prior to use. Expecting others to always leave it adjusted for your needs is rather selfish isn't it? If you must have a normalized setting, then putting both the seat and the lid down is the only fair solution under normal circumstances. However, when IBD is involved that's probably the worst option—when you're in a hurry that hole needs to be open already, one way or another. Leaving the lid up (preferably with the seat down) is a courteous favor that shortens the Nature 911 response time.

• *Toilet paper should roll off the top on the FRONT side of the roll.* Yeah I know there's some dissension on this one. A home-maker magazine once reported that this was their most common letter-to-the-editor topic. Google it. You'll be surprised how much collective brainpower has been spent on the debate over which way the TP should roll. The majority of internet polls lean in my favor. But come on, what's to debate? Rolling top to front makes the end closer and easier to see and reach.

• *Wiping should be done standing up, so there needs to be enough space for it.* Well maybe I'm a freak for this one—popular opinion tends to disagree with me on this issue, though the polls show winners both ways. I don't have any interest in shoving my hand through my crack and into the toilet bowl. Nope, not gonna happen, especially in a public restroom. Plus, squirming around on the pot increases the chances of inadvertently mopping the nasty front of the bowl with your pants. I'd rather leave that gunk behind, thank you. And finally, but most importantly, it allows you to observe what your body threw away before you cover it up, and with a disease like IBD, you gotta know. *Looking in the bowl helps you see inside the hole.*

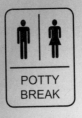

POTTY BREAK

So, while we're on the topic of bathrooms and sanitation, here's another seat cover story for you. This may sound very strange, but it's because of King Tut that I learned to make a toilet seat cover out of toilet paper. When I was seven years old, some family friends offered to take my brother and me to the Field Museum in Chicago to see the King Tut exhibit. It was the mid-seventies, and King Tut was a really big deal. Pop culture was obsessed with this Egyptian wonder. Steve Martin even wrote a song about it. It was a huge deal for us to go, and we were ecstatic about our museum day in the big city.

At some point, probably during the many hours waiting in line to get into the exhibit, I needed a potty stop. The friend of my folks took me into a stall and covered the seat with strips of TP so I didn't have to sit directly on it. I had never seen that done before, but it struck me as being pretty clever. Nowadays I still do it sometimes, but only when I'm feeling uneasy about the cleanliness of my locale. I'm generally far too rushed to spend time on that process, plus, when you have to use public restrooms everywhere, you eventually harden to such concerns.

In any case, I've been influenced by King Tut forever, in this one special way, and I'm pretty certain that's a unique relationship the Pharaoh doesn't share with anyone else.

But the seat cover saga doesn't end in ancient Egypt. Roman times have also made a contribution. As you might expect, this civilization offered me a more advanced technological solution.

My friend Tom is a goof ball. We worked together for a long time and were housemates for a couple years. We got into plenty of strange situations. He's been known to have a digestive issue or two now and then as well, so we can see eye-to-eye on the topic.

One time we were driving to Los Angeles together for work and decided to stop off in Vegas overnight. We got a few hours of sleep after a 24-hour drive, then explored The Strip before continuing on to L.A. At one point we were in Caesar's Palace looking for a bathroom. At that time, the bathrooms were located below the main casino floor, down an escalator leading to a lounge outside the restrooms. There were a lot of people there standing around, waiting for family members or whatever. I finished in the can first and waited in the lounge area for Tom. After a couple minutes he came out with a huge grin on his face. He was carrying a paper toilet-seat cover and holding it out to me. Loudly enough for everyone in the lounge to hear, he waved it around in the air and exclaimed,

"Here you go Andy, now you can say you got one from Caesar's Palace too!"

The looks we got were incredulous. Who the heck would collect toilet seat covers? We laughed all the way up the escalator and out the door.

To complete the story, years later I was back in Vegas again and made a point to get another seat cover from the same bathroom. I went to the cashier's window to see if they could help me authenticate that it came from Caesar's somehow. She let me use their check endorsement stamp to emboss the Caesar's Palace name on it. I put it in an envelope and mailed it to Tom without a note or return address. I'd have liked to be there when he opened it. I can't go to Vegas or see a toilet seat cover now without remembering and smiling about that silliness.

Flare-O-Gram

Yes, I've learned a lot about living with IBD over the past six years since my adventure began. My life is pretty good. But I don't mean to indicate that the challenges are over. Just about every week I face a new difficulty that reminds me I will be managing the inconvenience and anxiety of inflammatory bowel disease for the rest of my life. Here's a reminder that I experienced the other night—yes, even while I was almost finished with writing this book! Ugh, here we go again!

I wake up in the dark with a stomach ache. Even as I try to lie quietly, the pain increases. I get up. On the toilet I wrestle with last night's dinner. I return to bed nervous. What is going on? Was it disagreeable food? Is it the flu? Am I relapsing?

These wake-up calls happen periodically. Any time I feel digestive symptoms, they make me wonder and worry. If the symptoms are familiar they make me afraid that my colitis is flaring up. If they are unfamiliar, I can sometimes make myself believe that I have something unrelated like a cold or flu, which would be manageable (hopefully). But all too often these unfamiliar symptoms, especially the digestive ones, make me worry that my disease has progressed to a new level. I wonder if the disease has spread further or created additional complications. Or I fear that perhaps the strong medications have finally damaged my liver, pancreas, or another body system.

Once I am into this pattern of thinking I find very little comfort. I get nervous. The anxiety cycle kicks in, adding all of its sensations and fears. At least now I have learned to identify those, and I understand their role in my process. Nevertheless those times I wake, I lay in bed shivering, buzzing with troublesome thoughts. Instead of sleeping, I sweat. Instead of relaxing, I bundle into a fetal ball and tremble. Instead of getting rest, I fatigue. Eventually I succumb to exhaustion and finally fall asleep. I wake in the morning feeling unsettled and un-refreshed.

I get out of bed hoping that some water or food might help. The stomach ache seems to recede, but my concerns about it do not. I wonder. I lament. I worry. I call in sick and stay home from work. Often the trouble passes as I spend the day trying to relax. I watch a movie and have some comfort food. Periodically, during moments when my mind has been distracted from all the worry, I feel physically good and take a moment of pleasure in being home and comfortable. But then I remember that I'm actually sick and the reason I'm home relaxing is because I am experiencing something miserable.

This feeling is bad enough when I'm simply out of commission for a day or two, but when you consider how that emotional package overlays my entire life as an ever-present layer of chronic illness, you get an impression of how I experience the same "sick day" feeling about life in general. It hovers in the background all the time while I go about living my life.

This life-sized version hits me in a much bigger way than the simple tummy ache, however, and the weight can be oppressive. When I'm feeling well I often experience fun and joy, as one would hope. But at times even a small reminder of my permanent condition can temper the joy, not just on sick days, but every day. And so those indicators, however subtle, can be very discouraging. In essence I'm "home sick" every single day, however I feel and wherever I go. But I can't call in sick and stay home from life.

Belly cycles like the one I'm having at the moment have repeated themselves many times. Typically they're short lived—a minor bug or temporary flare-up. But this time it's a little different. Some of the discomfort seems more characteristically IBD-related, and it hasn't gotten better in the week since it started. Other symptoms are unfamiliar and therefore troubling. I call my doctor's office to move up my next regular GI appointment in case I am experiencing something that needs prompt attention. It troubles me to do this because it is an admission to myself that I might have something potentially serious to worry about. It's a reality check and I don't like it.

In this case, however, an interesting dynamic develops. I call and leave a message with the receptionist. Later I get a call back from a nurse, who then leaves a message for the scheduler, who will call me back later. While this process is typically frustrating, this time I find the complex sequence to be comforting in an unexpected way.

It makes me feel like I am approaching the difficult reality in small steps. I describe my symptoms to a nurse who listens calmly and seems to understand my predicament. By not insisting that I come in immediately, she insinuates that I'm probably OK at the moment. By waiting for the scheduler's callback I feel like I'm not making an immediate commitment and am therefore giving myself time to adjust to the idea before arranging an appointment. Then waiting a few days to get in also helps me adapt to the reality. Of course it will also take time to wait for lab test results afterwards. And this delay will allow me time to adjust to my doctor's impressions.

Like lying on a bed of nails, my emotional adjustments are broken up into many small points, which all together provide support that eventually leads me to feel a bit of comfort, despite my prickly situation. At the very least, scheduling an appointment makes me feel like I've done something proactive about my predicament.

The reality now is that I don't know what the diagnosis going to be. Maybe a flare, perhaps evidence of disease in new locations, maybe something else. The school year has just started again, so it's the most likely time for my wife and I to pick up viruses and other germs from students. But for practical reasons, it seems to be the worst possible time for this to happen. During the school year I have much more stress and much less flexibility in my schedule to accommodate office visits and whatever else impending illness or complications may bring—additional diagnostics, more tests, new medications, who knows. Plus I face that daily commute. What if symptoms make the long repetitive drive difficult or impossible;

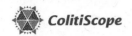

what will I do? There's plenty to be anxious about. I focus on trying to stay calm and keeping busy with useful activities that get me thinking about other things.

So what's next? It's hard to say in this case; time will tell. This is the life I live now. I feel well most of the time, but I experience occasional episodes that upset my delicate balance. Comfort and complacency come with stability, but when conditions change I quickly spring back to hypervigilant attention. Luckily, most of these episodes have been resolved favorably, either on their own or with minor adaptations to my diet or medications. The situation I'm in at the moment may also blow over without trauma. Or it may not.

Maybe it's time for new meds—Remicade or Humira. That solution would be a big change and is troublesome for its own reasons. Looking back on when my doctor confronted me with the suggestion that I switch to Remicade, I had lamented that there were no acute symptomatic catalysts urging me to do so. It makes me realize that I should be careful what I wish for, it might come true! Maybe now it has, or maybe not. Hopefully I will find out soon, or next time, or at some future date. This uncertainty is always with me, but as long as I'm feeling relatively well, I can maintain a state of equilibrium.

And, so goes my life with IBD—yes, even this very morning while I work to finish writing this book. It's an ongoing adventure that is manageable as a whole, but not without some bumps in the road.

Ice Hole

Before we close this book, I'd like to leave you with one more story—an anecdote that presents one of the dilemmas familiar to sufferers of all bowel-related ailments and perhaps shared by many other people. We've all had bathroom emergencies in strange circumstances, haven't we? Here is one last vivid glimpse of my life with digestive illness.

It was Christmas time again, exactly five years after my first colitis symptoms appeared on the flight to Rome. Heather and I had decided to venture north and spend time with old friends in the Midwest. Sure, winter is harsh up there, but we hadn't experienced the cold since we'd moved to the Southwest seven years earlier. What I was looking forward to most was participating in some of the outdoor winter activities I'd come to miss, as well as some that I'd never had the opportunity to do before. Our friends Anne and Shane had recently bought a pair of snowmobiles. They live in a farm town near a good sized lake—and that meant the possibility of limitless sledding and ice fishing.

The fun began the night we arrived. Shane had the snow machines ready to go. We got bundled up in several layers of wool, Thinsulate, nylon, cordura, and whatever else nature and man have come up with to allow us cold-weather recreation. I wouldn't

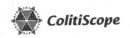

necessarily have chosen a nighttime ride for my first snowmobile experience, but I was not about to turn it down.

When I was young, adventures such as this were often spoiled by faulty machinery like my grandpa's old boat, which always promised a water-ski but then inevitably broke down while the first skier was dangling in the water waiting. Typically, in true irony, that poor disappointed brother, cousin, or self would end up tugging the crippled boat back to the dock with the water-ski rope.

I also have an older brother who rode everything first, sometimes breaking it on the maiden voyage, so I never got a chance. That happened with our go-kart, which we spent the remainder of the summer repairing and never riding.

With these debacles in mind, I remember pleading with Shane several times before our visit, "Just don't break them before I get there." After that kind of baggage with boy-toys, I was not about to miss an opportunity like this just because it was dark outside.

After an hour of loading the snowmobiles on the trailer, meeting up with Shane's two brothers, de-trailering the machines, getting the truck stuck in a snow bank, getting the truck un-stuck from a snow bank, waiting for Shane's brother to fix a broken bolt on his sled, etc., we finally fired them up and hit the snow. It was great, everything I had imagined it to be—exhilarating, nerve-racking, really cold, and just plain fun. Though Shane spent the rest of the week wincing in pain with every laugh because he was clever enough to roll his snowmobile while out on the lake that night. He glanced off a snow bank, and it sent him skidding off across the ice. All I got to see was the curlicue his lights made as the sled tumbled through the darkness. Shane had some fancy name for the rib cartilage he thought was damaged, but "ouchy-laugh" is close enough for me.

The next day was reserved for ice fishing. This quaint sacred ritual is a strange concept to most of the world. However, in northern Minnesota it is no different than summer fishing—or hunting, for that matter—it's all about equipment, accessories, and beer. People build fish houses out of whatever they can find and then haul them out onto a frozen lake as a sort of shelter while they fish and partake in other related activities. The less creative buy them ready-made with convenience features that degrade the true ice fishing experience. Homemade ice houses, on the other hand, are an intriguing combination of creativity, resourcefulness, and whimsy.

Shane's brothers Nate and Pat had one built of plywood and old trailer parts, which they could tow onto the lake like a trailer, then recess the wheels to the side allowing the structure to drop flat on the ice. The footprint was about six feet square. Inside it had a kerosene furnace, enough space for two overturned 5-gallon pails (the north woods Lay-Z-Boy) and two holes in the floor for fishing through the ice. The clever among you will notice that suspiciously missing from my description is a bathroom or porta-potty, hmmm.

These huts often have nameplates and addresses on the outside and decorations, racing stripes, murals, or whatever else helps builders claim them as their own creation. Just as popular fishing holes get busy with boats in the summer, these same spots get covered in winter with little cities of fish houses, complete with plowed roads, parking lots, and street signs. The first who dare the thin ice in the fall get to claim the prime spots. Everyone else fills in between trying to cash in on the better fishing. Solitude, however, is a big part of the ice fishing tradition, so the structures are always spaced at least a few dozen yards apart.

By the time Shane and I were mobilized for the long snowmobile trip to the lake, Nate and Pat had already set up their shack about a mile from shore near their parents' house, where it would stay for the remainder of the winter. They had borrowed Shane's truck to tow it out there, and in the back of the truck our fish tent was waiting. We made the five-mile snowmobile trek out to the ice town and found Shane's brothers toasty and warm, relaxing in their winter palace. They had their jackets off, showing waffle-textured long johns peeking out from under their flannel shirts.

My zipper thermometer showed minus seven degrees, and after racing through that frigid air at 40 mph on a snowmobile, I could definitely feel a chill. We unloaded Shane's hut from the truck. It was a more portable form of ice house, sort of a clever tent system that folds into a tub that you can drag around with a rope or tow with a snowmobile. We slid it out to a nice spot, drilled a couple holes with a power auger (can a Minnesota man really have fun without burning fossil fuels?) and set it up. It popped up like opening an umbrella, emerging from the tub into an eight-foot-square tent. We positioned it over the holes and sealed the bottom edges against the ice to keep out the wind. Inside, a bench seat folded out of the tub. We would sit on it while watching motionless bobbers for hours on end. It got dark as we finished setting up—at this latitude the late-December sun drops like a bowling ball at around 4:30.

We climbed inside, and Shane fired up the propane heater and a Coleman lantern hanging from the roof. We hooked a couple of minnows and dropped them into the holes using miniature two-foot fishing poles. These rods had built-in floor stands, so they could sit on the ice unattended. The heater cast a warm orange glow over the ice and our faces as we sat in quasi-darkness. Fifteen minutes seemed like forever.

As a truck drove by enroute to a neighboring hut, I could see the water oscillate up and down in the hole. The ice there was about a foot thick. I couldn't help but wonder how trial-and-error systems had determined ice safety over the years. The northlander-accented bait shop guys had reassured us that the lake had at least a foot of ice, plenty for trucks. "Sleds and four-wheelers only need six inches or so, don't cha knoow?" I shiver at the forbidden thought.

We focused on the motionless bobbers often enough for me to wonder what this was all about. *Oh yeah, now that we're done with the equipment it's time for the booze,* I reminded myself. Under normal circumstances, being stranded out in a place like this, eating and drinking would have been out of the question for me—but it was minus seven degrees outside; we had a giant thermos full of hot chocolate and Bailey's. And the beef sticks—it might be a guy thing, but as far as I am concerned they are worth the risk anywhere, any time. We had good fresh ones from a butcher shop, not the preservative-filled junk you find at the gas station. We chowed down, sipping warmth into our frigid bones. After snowmobiling across a lake and setting up this apparatus in these temperatures, we were definitely ready for it.

We sat chatting, trading stares between the glowing heater sitting on the ice in front of us and our bobbers, barely visible in the shadowed, watery holes. Eventually the inevitable time came; my gut began to grumble and groan, and I had to start up my personal panic-suppression machine. The trouble with feeling pretty well most of the time is that my preparatory discipline gets rusty. I don't always carry tissues and my mini-emergency kit. I get more ambitious about where I'll go without the certainty of restrooms and other protection. I'll eat beef sticks and drink hot chocolate in bad places. While this is a nice freedom, it doesn't always go smoothly (such as while ice fishing in the tundra with no emergency supplies).

I quietly considered my options. We rode out here on snowmobiles, and I was pretty sure I could find my way back to Shane's folks' house, but the trip would probably take more time than I could spare. And that was ignoring the tricky process of getting the engine started. After agonizing for a few minutes, I decided to share my predicament with Shane to see what sort of solutions we could come up with together. Shane had no napkins or tissues along. His truck was still attached to the fish house and probably wasn't convenient for a trip to shore (lest I drag his brothers for a joy ride), but it might contain some supplies. I got up to have a look.

By the time I unzipped and re-zipped the tent door, I had been vertical long enough to know that I was running low on time. I was also rudely reminded that minus seven is dang cold—actually since the sun went down, the temperature had dropped to minus twelve. I found my way to the truck, wasting precious time trying the passenger door first; it was locked. I went around to the driver's door and discovered that Shane's truck was clean as a whistle. All I found was a couple of helmets on the seat and his keys buzzing in the ignition. I lay over the seat to check the glove box. Empty. Not even an owner's manual. Bummer. I thought the first twenty pages of useless safety warnings might have sufficed nicely. It really was too bad the wind had blown all the snow off the ice, snowballs might actually have done the trick. I was really getting uncomfortable by then.

So I headed to the hut where his brothers were fishing for crappies, appropriately enough. I opened the door and felt the warmth flowing out on my face as I peered inside.

"Do you guys have any tissues, Kleenex, anything I can—"

"Need to make a man-pon?" Nate asked.

"Well, sort of, I gotta fish for the other kind of crappie, and it's a sure catch if you know what I mean."

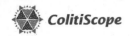

Chuckling, Pat replied, "Try my truck, there's probably something in there."

Remember, I was in Minnesota. Rural Minnesota. You need to understand something about the culture there before I tell you what I found in that truck. Everybody remembers when Pat got married because they held it on Fishing Opener, the first weekend of fishing season. This is a state where, when Mother's Day occasionally coincides with Fishing Opener, they have a great debate about which so-called holiday to reschedule. Suffice it to say folks showed true love by making it to the wedding. It's a good thing they didn't have it on first weekend of deer hunting season though; they'd have walked down the aisle of an empty church.

Anyway, I checked the glove box, the center console and the floor all around the front seats. I found no paper, save for two crumpled fast food napkins under the front seat—I eagerly claimed my new prize, it was a good start but not enough. The naked lady playing cards on his key chain looked promising until I realized they were stiff plastic. I decided to search the back seat for forgotten remnants of meals on the road or whatever I might find. I would have settled for an old t-shirt at that point. Instead what I encountered was a bewildering array of Minnesota stuff: half-empty boxes of three different ammo calibers, binoculars, a case for a different pair of binoculars, a couple of bobbers…all hidden under the clumsy pile of two rifles, a shotgun, their cases, a fishing pole and a handgun case. It was like a big boy's toy box dumped out on the floor. I dug farther under the seats and found another gun, a tree saw, matches, some boots, a bag of frozen Milk Duds, and a bunch of other stuff he probably forgot he had, but no paper products.

I remember the Boy Scout motto "be prepared." Well, with access to this pickup truck I had sufficient supplies to build a fire and feed myself by land or sea like Daniel Boone, enough armaments to invade Canada (which, conveniently enough, could be reached from here with the gas remaining in my snowmobile), and plenty of frozen candy to break all the teeth on all of the crazy fishermen on the lake that night—but I was left completely unprepared for the simple task of taking a dump.

I paused for a tense moment to survey my situation. It was getting more urgent. I had the napkins, but two wipes would certainly not be enough. No way. I kicked around at the ice below me, too crusty to muster up any snowballs. My only other option seemed to be pounding across a mile of frozen drifts on a snowmobile. At that point there was absolutely no way I could have managed that without popping.

I headed back toward the tent. My face was beyond stinging and mostly numb. I remarked to myself again how absurdly cold it was and how insane a person would have to be to try this so-called sport more than once.

I climbed back inside and asked Shane again what provisions we had. We took a full inventory of the tent house and discovered nothing useful. For a moment I considered the leaf wrapper of the cigar he was smoking, but thought better of suggesting it. He sorted through the garbage and all he could come up with was an empty M&Ms wrapper with some sort of slimy goo on the outside. I inspected it in the light of the lantern and reluctantly decided that I might stand a chance with a third resource.

"Better use that one first," Shane cleverly advised as I unzipped the door and went back out.

Then I had to face the question of where I could actually go to take care of business. I couldn't really squat behind a fish house because there were people in all of them. One thing in my favor was that people had been ice fishing all over out there so I found dozens of holes in the ice, just waiting for me, though I knew I'd better not stay too close lest my by-product come up as unwanted game for a fishermen nearby. Plus, Pat and Nate had a fish finder; they'd have a perfect sonar view of my turds sinking to the bottom. Now that would have provided a story for the ages. The tent was far too permeable to offer any auditory camouflage, so I determined that I had to go out in the middle of the lake where nobody would see me on this cold, dark night, and where nobody would encounter my remains.

I walked about fifty yards into the dark oblivion and selected a hole that seemed as good as any other. I poked the toe of my boot into it. There was a thin sheet of ice covering the opening, which I broke loose hoping that by some miracle my refuse would land on target and disappear to the depths below. The hole provided a ten-inch opening, significantly smaller than the diameter of a standard toilet, and I wasn't exactly shooting from point-blank range. Mind you, the last full moon was two weeks past; all I could really see were the glowing windows in the fish houses littering the lake-scape. As I struggled to see evidence of the lake shore in the distance, the howling wind made my eyes water, painting ice-cold lines on my cheeks.

This task was going to require some careful planning. I surveyed my supplies, peeling open the candy wrapper, hoping for a cleaner interior. It was definitely cleaner than the exterior, but also coated in the same glossy plastic layer as the outside. It would have to do; there was no way I could do the job without it. The wrapper would come first, followed by the two napkins. I carefully folded each so that I could easily reverse the fold and use them a second time.

Complicating matters further, I was bundled up like the Michelin Man. I was wearing an undershirt, turtleneck, vest, and heavy jacket, not to mention a knit face mask and fur hat that I could barely see out of—and that's only what I had on above the waist. I was going to have to do my business without freezing to death, but it became obvious that there was no way I could manage with the parka on, so I took it off and carefully laid it on the ice with the inside facing up so it didn't collect ice or snow, putting my gloves on top. The wind chill was minus twenty; I was shivering instantly. I meticulously arranged the precious papers in my vest pockets to be sure they'd be readily accessible from my compromised squatting position. The snot was already dripping from my frozen nose. At this temperature, I was surprised the drips didn't freeze the moment they surfaced.

Finally I felt sufficiently staged for my coordinated mission; there was only one thing left to do, and it wasn't gonna be pleasant. I backed up to the hole and dropped my drawers. Now that seems like a simple enough task, but realize that on the bottom I was wearing underwear, long johns, jeans and snow bib overalls. This was not an easy process, but I'll spare you the details because they alone would occupy a couple of extra pages. It took a lot of work, but I finally got everything down, being careful not to dangle the bib shoulder straps in the wrong places, and with relief I finally let 'er rip.

I already knew it was cold out there, but now that my warmest parts were dangling over an icy hole in the middle of a mile-wide lake that had been frozen for two months, I started to appreciate what it truly means to live in this climate. I had a hard time squatting with the three pairs of pants bundled around my knees, and really didn't want to miss, so I was relieved to hear the muffled splashes in the hole behind me—actually shocked that I even got close. After taking a moment to be sure it was all done, I felt relieved.

It was quite peaceful out there, I must admit, and surprisingly private. Or so I thought until my solitude was rudely interrupted by the headlights of a pickup truck about a hundred yards away. They weren't pointing directly at me, but I was certainly in their path; I could see my shadow on the ice. *Can they even see this far?* I wondered. Regardless, I panicked and shifted my efforts to make a hasty cleanup—so hasty in fact that all my careful planning went right out the window. The slippery M&M wrapper was nearly useless, missed the hole, and went fluttering off in the wind. The two napkins supplied only a single use each despite my master plan to the contrary, and were dropped indiscriminately as my clumsy pants-system came up, at best slightly prematurely. Then, as abruptly as it had illuminated the scene, the pickup truck turned away, suddenly leaving me in the dark again.

I wondered for a moment whether the napkins could be retrieved for another use, but once my eyes re-adjusted to the darkness, I realized that despite my haste they had landed directly in the hole and were already starting to freeze into the icy surface of the water a foot down. I kicked whatever crust and snow I could muster into the hole and hoped it would freeze over and disappear until spring when I'd be long gone.

Some hand sanitizer would have been really nice right about then, but the best I could do was find a fresh fishing hole and splash my hands in it. A shudder ripped through my body as I realized that the water was literally freezing cold. Duh! First, instantaneous shooting pain, then utter numbness. I shook my hands in the wind and let out an unconscious hoot as I buried them deep in my vest pockets to warm them up. I picked up my parka which had been in a deep freeze for several minutes by then. The stiff fabric was a precursor to the cruel frigidity of putting it on. Operating the zipper proved rather clumsy because my hands were so cold my fingers felt like dead stumps. I hopped around a few times, freezing, trying to fathom what could have possessed me to do this. Now that the hot chocolate was gone, our snack no longer seemed to have been worth the risk, though at that particular point I would have drunk it again just to feel the warm cup on my hands. I made my way back to the tent and welcomed the only-slightly-warmer air inside.

Then the real gamble began. I had already used up whatever make-shift supplies I could find, so if my colon mustered up another episode, I would really be up a creek—the one and only kind of "creek." I hated to end the party, so I sat for a while longer before breaking the news to Shane. We'd have to pack it up pretty soon. We agreed to leave in a half hour if there was still no action. That was reassuring because the nil chances of me actually encountering any fishing action have been proven time and again over many years. Then it occurred to me, I had a fishing license in my pocket; it was made of paper! I could have used that. It turned out I certainly didn't need it for fishing. It could have been the best twenty-five bucks I'd ever spent.

My nervous wait ended early when Nate came by to announce he was heading ashore to bring Pat's wife out for some fishing. It was the perfect catalyst for us to bail out due to the complex vehicle logistics involved. We packed up the tent much faster than it went up, stashed it in the truck, started our snowmobiles, and headed for the shoreline.

Later, after Shane's brothers returned from their much warmer fish house, Pat recalled their participation in my little adventure. You need to appreciate the thick, *Fargo*-esque, Minnesota accent to get the true picture.

"Just after Andy came in looking for shit tickets, Nate asked me, 'Is he really gonna take a dookie out on the ice?'"

"Yep, I think so."

"Geez, I hope I don't step in it."

Shit tickets? Seriously, that's the funniest thing I've heard in a long time. Who came up with that? Doesn't matter, it's my new favorite word anyway. And I'm definitely bringing some along the next time I go ice fishing—which will be, well, probably never.